D0319783

THE BRAID BOOK

20 FUN AND EASY STYLES

SARAH HISCOX & WILLA BURTON
OF THE BRAID BAR

PHOTOGRAPHY BY JESSE JENKINS

KYLE BOOKS

CONTENTS

BRAIDS 30

I N T R O

Braids are like leopard print — sometimes they're in but they're never out! Let's face it, braids rule and we love a good braid! They're popular because they have the ability to complete a look. Braids are way more interesting and edgy than a blow-dry, and there are so many styles to choose from. They can also be incredibly helpful if you're working non-stop for a week and you don't want to worry about what your hair looks like.

Here are some answers to questions we always get asked by our braid fans. It's the official top 10 FAQs for all things braid!

1. HOW DID YOU COME UP WITH THE NAMES OF THE BRAIDS? We named our styles after well-known supermodels and other influential women that most girls would recognise. These women are all strong and much more than a pretty face. They are determined women who have succeeded in a multitude of roles.

2. WHAT IS YOUR MOST POPULAR BRAID? The most popular is definitely the Cara 2.0 or the Kate. Apart from being named after our two most famous style icons, they are both great looks! They're very cool and I think girls quite like the idea of being able to have a braid and keep their hair down at the same time.

3. WHAT IS YOUR FAVOURITE BRAID? Sarah: I LOVE the Cara 2.0 as it's a braid that definitely suits everyone! I prefer braids where I can have my hair down as well, so this style ticks all the boxes. It's really edgy without making too much of a statement. Willa: The Tyra is my fave – I love the idea that you can do something to totally change your look but can take it out the next day! You can never be bored with a braid!

4. WHAT'S THE SIMPLEST BRAID? Definitely the Gisele. The beauty of the Fishtail braid is that it looks really complicated but it's not! Friends will be so impressed by it but you don't have to tell them how easy it was. It's our secret, right?

5. WHICH IS THE BEST BRAID FOR… A WEDDING? The Claudia or the Gisele.

They are both very pretty and feminine and look stunning if you wind fresh flowers into the braids. It's a really natural, beautiful look.

…A JOB INTERVIEW? The Claudia or the Linda – they're smart and sassy and look like you mean business!

…A NIGHT OUT? The Carla or the Tyra – they give you a completely different look. They definitely say wild and fun!

…A FIRST DATE? The Kate or the Cara 2.0 – they're really sexy but you're keeping it feminine and they don't look like you've made too much of an effort!

…A FESTIVAL? The Gwen! It's perfect for that fest-vibe. Really go mad and add rings, feathers, chalks and glitter – think more, more, more!

6. HOW LONG DO THE BRAIDS LAST? The tighter the braids are, the longer they will last. For example, the Gwen or the Eva will probably last a week. See Caring for your Braid on page 18 for tips on how to make your braid last longer.

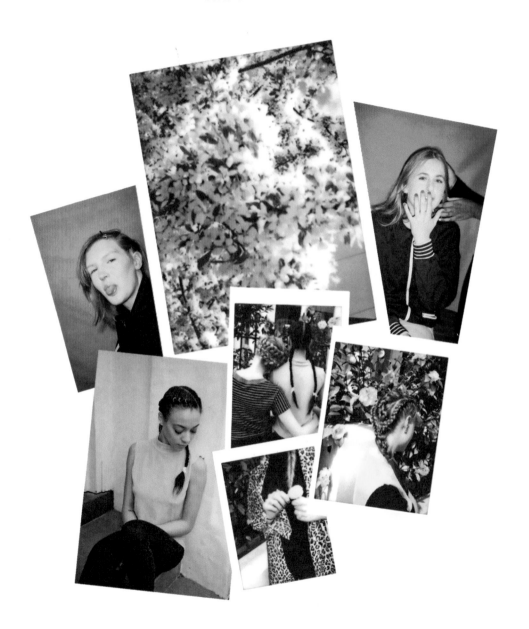

7. WHAT TYPE OF BRAID IS BEST FOR… THIN HAIR?

You can either tease thin hair before you start braiding to give it some depth or buy hair wefts from specialist hair salons that you can clip into your existing hair to make it look thicker and longer. We use coloured hair wefts which look amazing (see page 19)!

…GREASY HAIR? If you have greasy hair and can't be bothered to wash it, the best braids are the styles that use all the hair. Greasy hair is much easier to braid, so it's a win-win situation!

…SHORT HAIR? We get loads of girls (and boys) with bob haircuts or shorter who want to have braids. The most popular is the Eva as it works on any length hair.

8. CAN ANYONE BRAID?

Yes, everyone can be a Braid Babe! If you start off with the standard styles (French and Dutch on pages 22–25) and really practise them, then there is no braid you won't be able to master. Just keep practising!

After a lot of practice, you'll be able to do all of these braids yourself. But in the mean time, get a helping hand from a friend.

9. CAN YOU ACCESSORISE BRAIDS?

You can put anything you like in them. That's the beauty of braiding — they are so versatile. We like to hang hair rings and charms off our braids, as well as colouring them with chalk and glitter. Go wild and experiment.

10. WHAT ELSE CAN I DO WITH BRAIDS?

Have a party! We love to get our mates round and practise different styles on each other — it's such a laugh and you end up inventing brand new mad styles!

THE
ESSENTIAL
TOOL
KIT

CROCODILE CLIPS
Any pharmacy or hair shop will have some of these.

ELASTIC HAIR BANDS – CLEAR AND COLOURED
Pharmacies and high-street stores will stock these.

FINE-TOOTHED PINTAIL COMB
Pick one of these up from your local pharmacy.

HAIR SLIDES AND PINS (BLONDE AND DARK)
Try your local pharmacy or hair shop for these.

NORMAL HAIR BANDS
Any pharmacy or hair shop will have some of these.

PRÊT-À-POWDER (OR DRY SHAMPOO)
Great for oily hair or hair that has missed a wash or two! We like Bumble and Bumble's Prêt-à-Powder, which combines dry shampoo, style extender and a pinch of volume. Alternatively, you can use regular dry shampoo.

PRIMING SPRAY
Priming your hair before you braid is essential. Many primers have setting agents which will keep your braid neater for longer, the hair is also easier to work with when a little damp. Alternatively, use conditioner mixed with a bit of water.

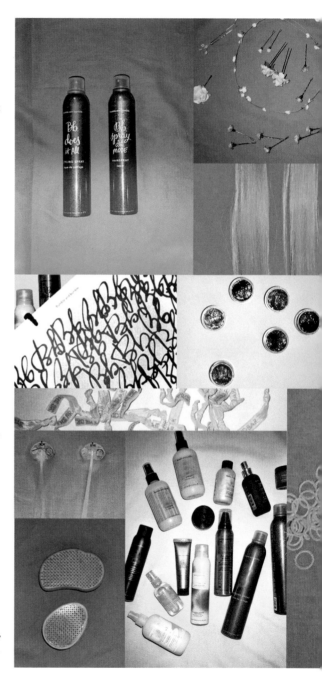

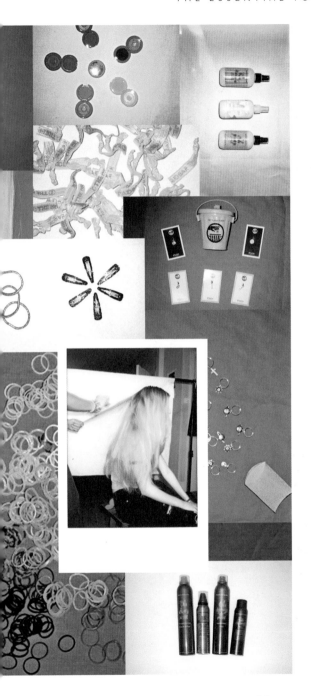

SALT SPRAY
Nowadays, many brands stock texturising salt sprays, but the original Surf Spray was made by Bumble and Bumble in 2001. It adds body and a matte finish. Available in selected stores and online.

STRONG-HOLD HAIRSPRAY
You can find this everywhere. Go for one that brushes out easily, such as L'Oreal, or adds texture and creates instant fullness, such as Bumble and Bumble's DrySpun Finish. Or look for one specific to your hair type.

VOLUMISING SPRAY
A thickening hairspray is worth investing in, especially if you have thin hair or just want to get some extra oomph. Tresemmé do a great one of these.

FINISHING SPRAY
You can find this in most pharmacies and online.

WIDE-TOOTHED COMB OR HAIRBRUSH
We like to use the world-famous Tangle Teezer.

HAIR CHALK
Sold in high street shops and online. Rub onto hair for a temporary colour fix.

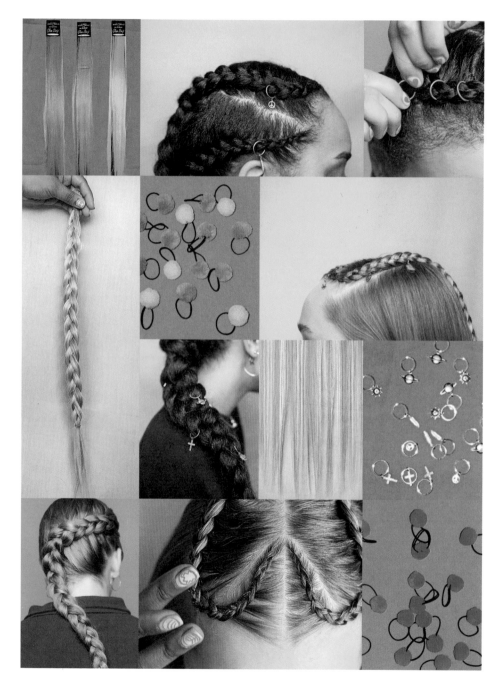

COLOURED HAIR STRIPS

Glam Strips by Manic Panic. www.manicpanic.com

FLOWERS

 Etsy shop 'BabyBunheads' make beautiful handmade
flowers. www.etsy.com

PLAIN BANDS
& GLITTER BANDS

Stocked at The Braid Bar. www.thebraidbar.co.uk

LED LIGHT STRIPS

Available on Amazon. www.amazon.co.uk

MY FLASH TRASH CHARMS

Made in Chelsea's Amber Atherton has her own
jewellery company, My Flash Trash. Check out her
adorable charms (page 13), perfect to add to your
braid for special occasions. www.myflashtrash.com

POMPOMS

Available from PomPom Galore.
www.pompomgalore.co.uk
You can also buy fluoro pompoms from
www.thebraidbar.co.uk

REGAL ROSE RINGS
& REGAL ROSE RING CHARMS

Stocked at The Braid Bar. www.thebraidbar.co.uk

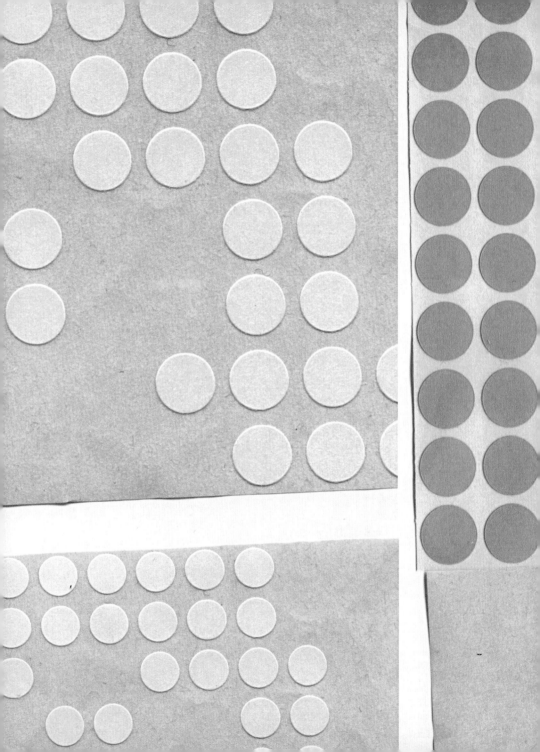

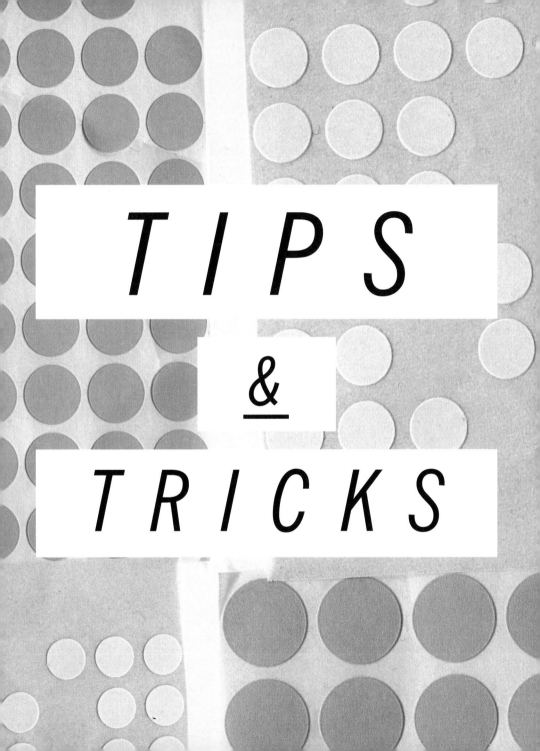

TIPS & TRICKS

CARING FOR YOUR BRAID

TO KEEP YOUR BRAID FRESH TO DEATH CHECK OUT SOME OF OUR TIPS AND TRICKS...

- Use a priming spray and finishing spray on your braid to ensure it sets well.

- At night, wrap a silk scarf around your head to prevent friction with the pillow.

- In the morning, reapply hairspray or any other finishing sprays.

- When in the shower, wash the hair around the braids, avoiding vigorous movements.

- If you are prone to greasy hair and you normally wash your hair once a day, use a little baby powder or dry shampoo. We like to use Bumble and Bumble's Pret-à-Powder — a translucent powder that acts as a dry shampoo and a volumiser at once!

- For very curly hair, sometimes it is good to give the hair a straightening blow-dry with a paddle brush before braiding.

- You can wash your braids, as long as they are tight — cornrows are no problem, but the bigger braids won't stay in.

WEAVE & WEFTS

IS YOUR HAIR TOO SHORT…? TOO FINE…? TOO THIN…?

Becoming a Braid Babe isn't always easy, you might be in need of some weave! You can clip it in, snip it off, dye it and tie it but most importantly you can braid it and no one would ever know it isn't your real hair! You can even use coloured weave to create that dip-dye effect without harming your own precious locks.

Weave is cheaper than semi-permanent extensions and can be found online or in your nearest African-Caribbean hair shop. There are hundreds of shades and textures, so it's your job to find the hair that is nearest to your own!

BASIC INSTRUCTIONS

STEP 1 Find the right shade and texture, and make sure the length of weave is longer than your own hair.

STEP 2 Clip it in before you braid or, if the hair is loose, simply add it in as you braid.

STEP 3 If you can get your hands on some feathering scissors, use these to give a realistic effect when cutting the hair to length.

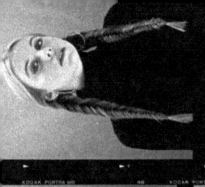
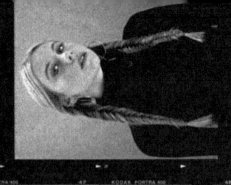
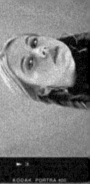

KODAK PORTRA 400   46   KODAK PORTRA 400   47   KODAK PORTRA 400   48   KODAK PORTRA 400

BASIC

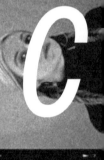

K PORTRA 400   50   KODAK PORTRA 400   51   KODAK PORTRA 400

BRAIDS

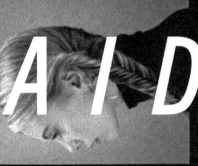
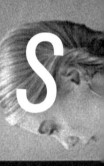

AK PORTRA 400   53   KODAK PORTRA 400   54   KODAK PORTRA 400

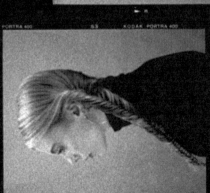
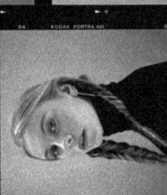

THE BASIC BRAID TYPES

FRENCH AND DUTCH BRAIDS, LACE AND FOUR-STRAND… WE'VE ALL ASKED OURSELVES THE SAME QUESTION: WHAT IS THE DIFFERENCE?

WE ARE HERE TO SHOW HOW TO DO THEM ALL, AS CLEARLY AND SIMPLY AS POSSIBLE!

YOU WILL NEED...

Wide-toothed comb or hairbrush
Priming spray
Fine-toothed pintail comb
Elastic bands
Hairspray

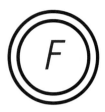

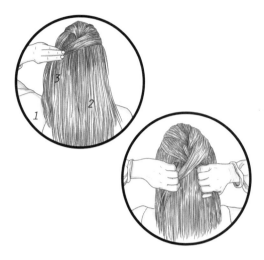

STEP 1 Begin by taking a section of hair from the top of the head at the hairline. Separate this section into three strands. Mentally label them 1, 2 and 3.

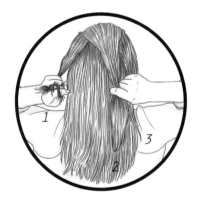

STEP 2 Cross the right strand (no. 3) over the middle strand (no. 2) and then the left strand (no. 1) over the new middle strand (no. 3). Keeping the strands separated, transfer all three into your left hand.

STEP 3 Using your right hand, grab a small section of hair from your right side and add to the right strand.

STEP 4 Now, bring that right strand over the middle strand and cross the middle strand over to the right. Keeping the strands separated, transfer all three strands into your right hand.

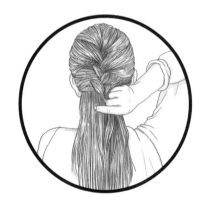

STEP 5 Repeat the process, adding small sections of hair from each side and cross the

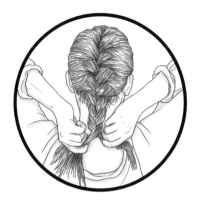

strands over as you would in a basic braid.

STEP 6 Finish the style with a basic braid and secure with an elastic band.

TIP Try to keep your hands as close to the head as possible to ensure a tight braid.

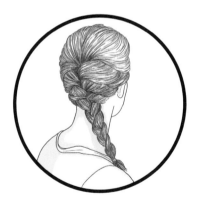

ESTIMATED TIME
15 mins

FRENCH

BRAID

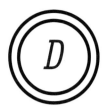

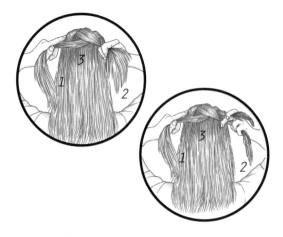

STEP 1 Begin by taking a section of hair from the top of the head. Separate this section into three strands. As before, label these strands 1, 2 and 3.

STEP 3 Now, with strand 2 you need to gather some loose hair to add to the braid (see above right illustration).

STEP 4 Before braiding in the new bit of hair — you must braid strand 1 under strand 3, then add some loose hair to strand 3. So now you should have strand 3 (plus added bit of hair) in your fingers, strand 1 in the middle, and strand 2 on the right hand side with some extra hair.

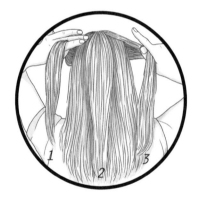

STEP 2 Pull the middle strand (no. 2) over the right strand of hair (no. 3) — this is the difference between the Dutch and French braids. Strand 2 is now the right strand and strand 3 is now the middle strand.

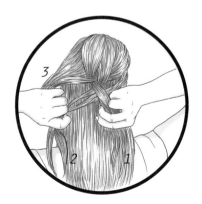

STEP 5 You now have to slowly take strand 1 above strand 2, making sure you keep hold of the extra hair you added in Step 3.

STEP 6 You then add extra hair to strand 1, which will now be on the right hand side, so it is ready for when you have braided the extra hair into the braid from the left.

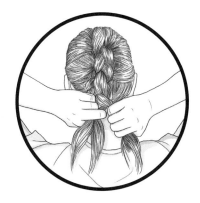

STEP 7 The next stage is to repeat what you have just done but now using the middle strand and the strand on the left hand side. So what you

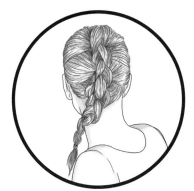

do is take the middle strand above the left strand making sure you keep hold of the extra hair and then add hair to the strand that is now on the left, as in steps 2–3.

STEP 8 Keep repeating these actions, making sure that you are adding hair with every move.

STEP 9 Finish with a basic braid and secure with an elastic band.

....

THE DUTCH BRAID IS A SIMILAR TECHNIQUE TO THE FRENCH BRAID, EXCEPT WHEN YOU ADD HAIR YOU CROSS THE STRAND UNDER THE BRAID RATHER THAN OVER.

ESTIMATED TIME
15 mins

DUTCH BRAID

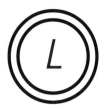

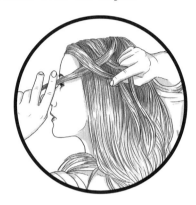

STEP 2 Start your braid by crossing the right strand over the middle and then the left strand over the right.

STEP 1 Take a section of hair and divide it into three strands.

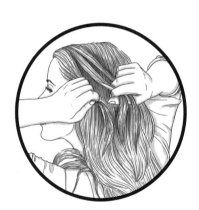

STEP 3 This braid is done using the French braiding technique but only adding hair from one side of the braid.

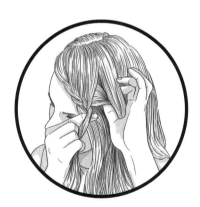

STEP 4 Angle the braid in the direction that you want it to go.

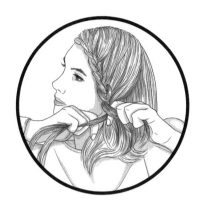

STEP 5 Repeat the French braiding technique adding small sections of hair as you go.

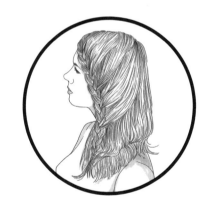

ESTIMATED TIME
15 mins

L
A
C
E

B
R
A
I
D

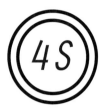

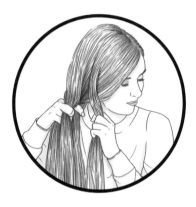

STEP 2 Start with the strand furthest away from the face as strand 1. Pull this over strand 2 and pull strand 3 over strand 4. Then pull strand 4 over strand 1.

STEP 1 Begin with four strands of hair. Number the strands 1 to 4 to keep them clear in your mind.

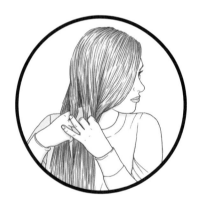

STEP 3 Renumber for each braid sequence. Remember: 1 over 2, 3 over 4, 4 over 1.

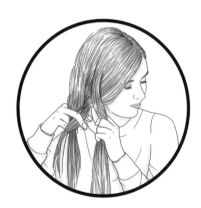

STEP 4 Repeat all the way
down and tie with a hair tie.

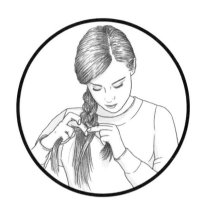

STEP 5 To see the intricate
braiding work, pull the braid
out a bit to flatten it. Finish
with hairspray.

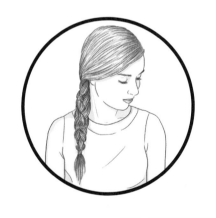

ESTIMATED TIME
15 mins

FOUR STRAND

BRAID

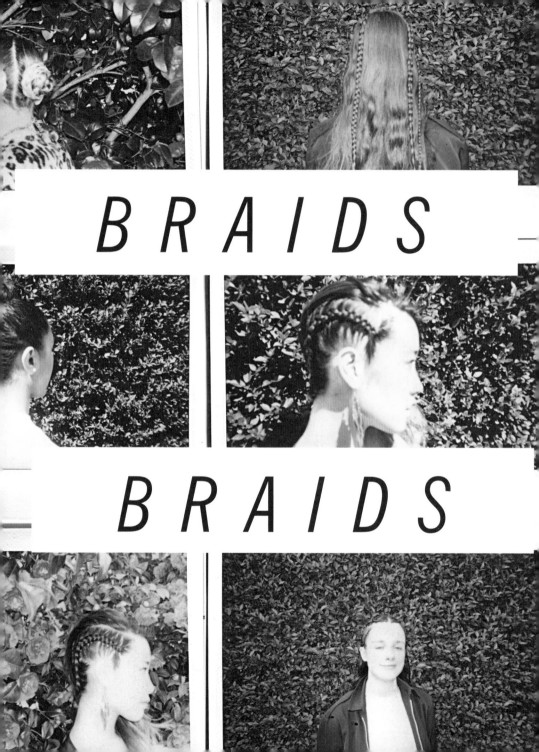

BRAIDS

BRAIDS

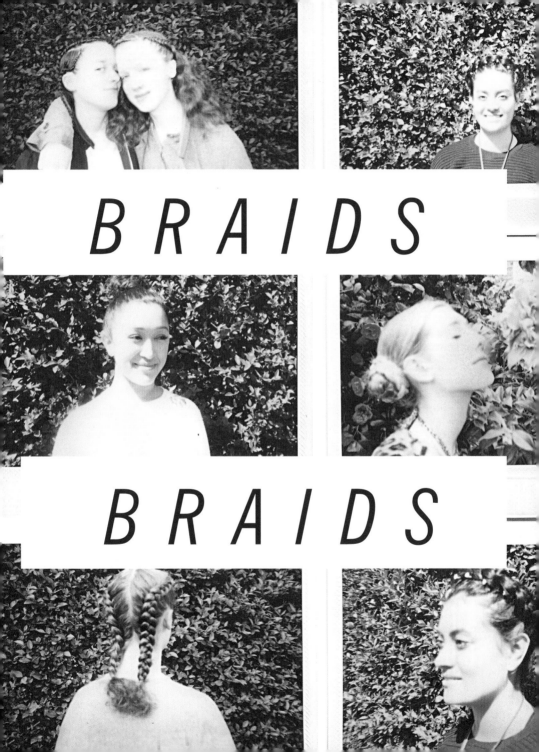

BRAIDS

BRAIDS

R 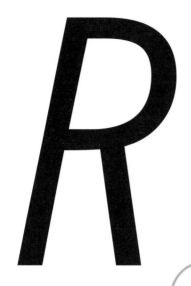 I

'AS A TEENAGE
LONG-DISTANCE
RUNNER
I FRENCH-
PLAITED MY HAIR
EVERY DAY FOR
AERODYNAMIC
EASE. ON
HOLIDAY I SLEEP
IN PLAITS AND
WAKE UP TO
WAVES. AND
NOW THAT
MY HAIR IS
RAPUNZEL-STYLE
TO MY WAIST,
I BRAID IT

R 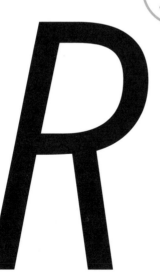 I

CENTRE-PARTED
HIAWATHA STYLE,
SOMETIMES
ROUGHLY PINNED
UP INTO A
TWISTED CROWN.
SPEED-FREAK
FREE-SPIRITED
STYLE FOR TOWN
OR COUNTRY;
BEAUTY AND
THE BEACH..'

—

LAURA BAILEY
(MODEL
& MOTHER)

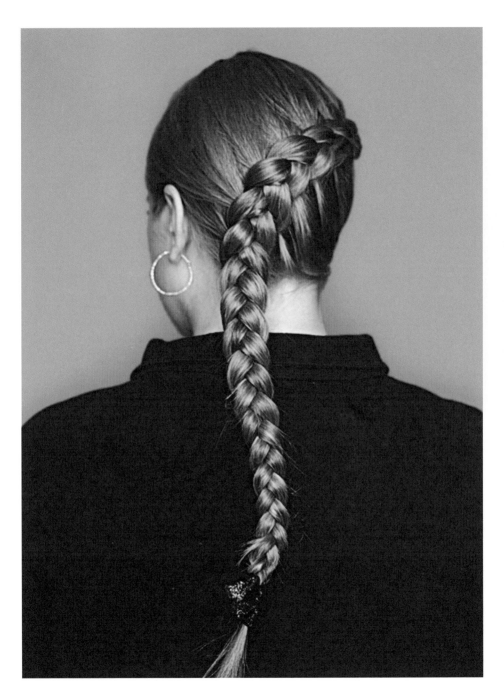

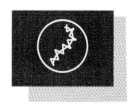

A TWIST ON THE BASIC DUTCH BRAID.

This braid is perfect for Dutch braid beginners as you can really put your newly acquired skills into action. We named this after Rihanna because she rocked something similar to the Met Ball a few years back.

YOU WILL NEED:
Wide-toothed hairbrush
Priming spray
Fine-toothed pintail comb
Elastic hair band

STEP 1 Detangle the hair and spritz with primer.

STEP 2 The braid begins from the side of the head, so choose which side suits you or your friend best.

STEP 3 Using your pintail comb, make a deep side parting on the side opposite to the one you've chosen. Begin the parting from directly above the beginning of your eyebrow.

STEP 4 Pull all your hair from the parting over to the opposite side and begin to Dutch braid (pages 24—25) with three strands, adding hair as you go.

STEP 5 Continue the braid, steering it diagonally across the back of the head creating an 'S' shape as you go.

STEP 6 At the nape of the neck, continue with a plain plait and secure with an elastic band.

    #THERIRIBRAID

STEP 1

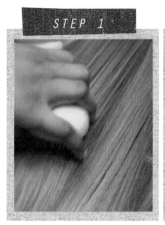

STEP 3

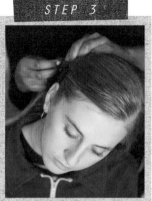

STEP 4

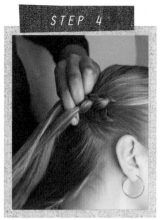

STEP 5

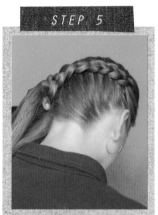

STEP 6

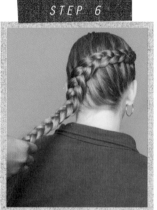

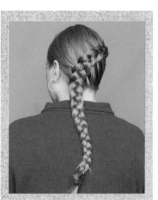

TIP

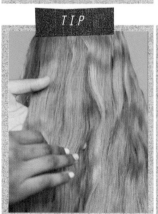

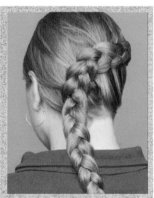

TIP This braid may seem a bit dull, so why not spice it up with some temporary colour using hair chalk. See page 13 for details.

THIS IS THE PERFECT GOING OUT
HAIRSTYLE, PARTICULARLY IF YOU HAVEN'T
HAD TIME TO WASH IT. INSPIRED BY THE
GREAT PARISIAN CARLA BRUNI, THIS STYLE
IS TRES CHIC AND TRES EASY ALSO!

CARLA

*'THE BRAID BAR IS EFFORTLESSLY COOL... IT'S THE
PLACE WHERE GANGS OF KIDS WANT TO GO... AND THEY
MADE ME FEEL AMAZING AT THE BAFTAS... LOVE THEM!'
DAVINA MCCALL (PRESENTER)*

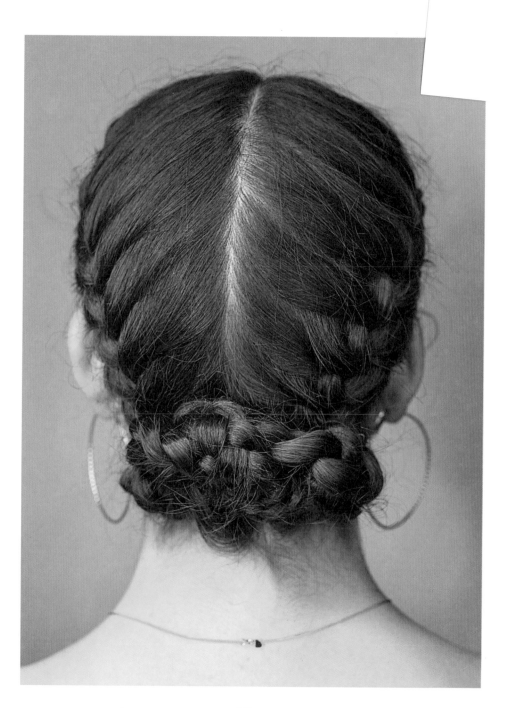

YOU WILL NEED:
Wide-toothed comb
  or hairbrush
Fine-toothed
  pintail comb
Crocodile clips
Bristle brush
Hairgrips
Elastic bands

STEP 1 Detangle the hair and spritz with primer.

STEP 2 Use your pintail comb to create either a centre or deep side parting, depending on what you would rather. Take it right down to your neck and clip one half of your hair out of the way.

STEP 3 Begin with one side and French braid (pages 22–23) as normal, adding hair as you go. Continue all the way down to the end of your hair.

TIP No need to make these braids really tight. Leave them slightly looser to create that messy-chic look. You may even want to go over it with a bristle brush.

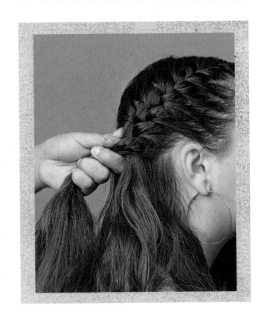

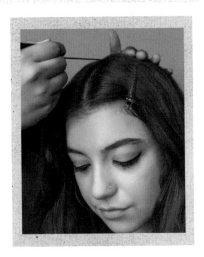

STEP 4 Secure the braid with an elastic band.

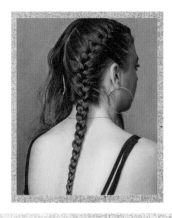

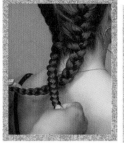

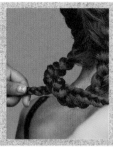

STEP 5 Repeat the process with the other half of your hair.

STEP 7 Repeat Step 6 and FINI!

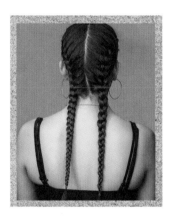

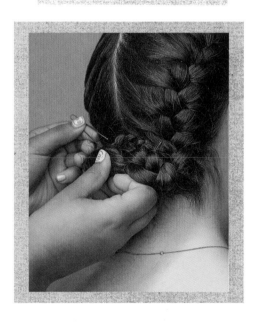

STEP 6 Take both braids and tie them together as if you were tying your shoe laces. Use lots of hairgrips and pin this into place.

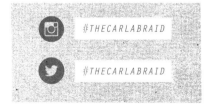

#THECARLABRAID

#THECARLABRAID

*YOU CAN GUESS WHICH STAR THIS
BRAID IS NAMED AFTER... THIS IS THE
BRAID BAR'S TAKE ON THE CLASSIC
'DOUBLE DUTCH' BRAIDS.*

The side parting used in this braid is
what will transform you from your average
babe to a braid babe! One of the easiest,
quickest and trendiest braids on our menu,
designed to make you feel as tough and
sexy as Naomi Campbell.

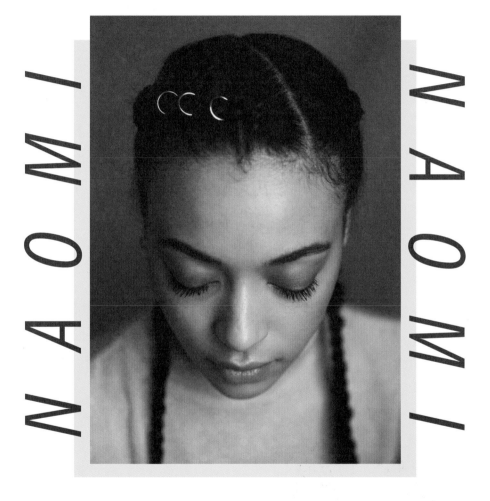

NAOMI

NAOMI

YOU WILL NEED:
Wide-toothed comb
 or hairbrush
Priming spray
Fine-toothed pintail comb
Small elastic hair bands
Volumising spray

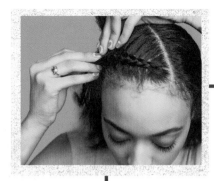

STEP 1 Detangle
the hair and spritz
with primer.

STEP 2 Using your
pintail comb, begin
the parting directly
above the outer end of
your eyebrow. Part the
hair in a curved shape,
diagonally across the
crown. Continue the
curve all the way to
the nape of the neck,
bringing it back to
the centre.

STEP 4 Begin Dutch
braiding (pages 24–25)
the first half of your
hair, following the
curve of your head
and continuing around
your ear.

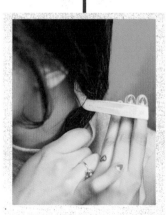

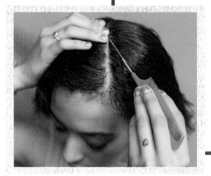

STEP 3 Tie one half of
your hair out of the way.

STEP 5 After braiding along the scalp and down to the nape of your neck, continue the braid to the end of your hair and tie using an elastic band.

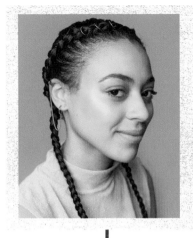

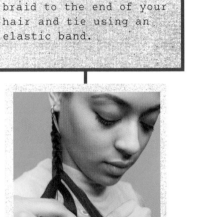

STEP 8 As a final touch, use a finishing volumising spray to keep this badass braid as clean and tidy as possible.

STEP 7 Repeat the exact same process with the other half of your hair. Remember that one half may be thicker than the other because they have not been parted equally.

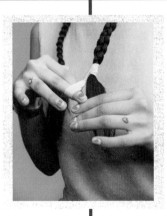

HAIR RINGS: At The Braid Bar we sell the fabulous Regal Rose Aeon Hair Rings. They come in silver and gold and bring a bit of punk to any look. We think they work on The Naomi the best.

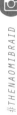

#THENAOMIBRAID #THENAOMIBRAID

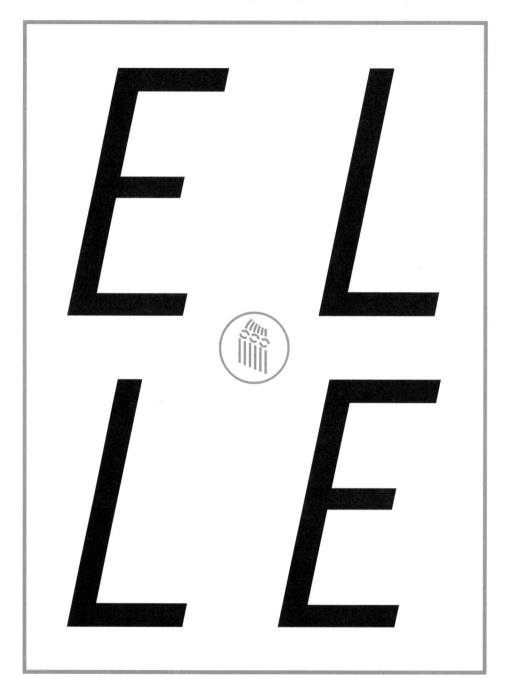

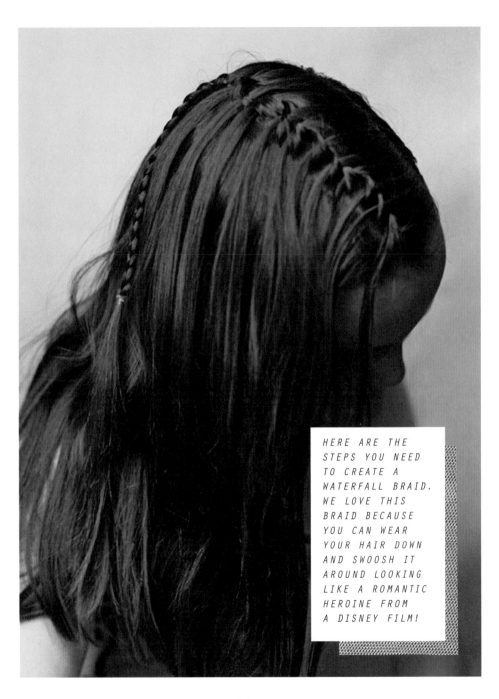

HERE ARE THE
STEPS YOU NEED
TO CREATE A
WATERFALL BRAID.
WE LOVE THIS
BRAID BECAUSE
YOU CAN WEAR
YOUR HAIR DOWN
AND SWOOSH IT
AROUND LOOKING
LIKE A ROMANTIC
HEROINE FROM
A DISNEY FILM!

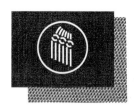

IT'S NAMED THE 'ELLE' BECAUSE IT PERFECTLY COMBINES THE VIBES OF QUEEN ELSA (FROZEN) AND ELLE MACPHERSON'S GORGEOUSNESS. Once you've mastered the basics of how to do it, you can use it in so many ways — tie it up into a pony, leave it loose or pull it into a messy bun. If you can do a French braid you should be able to master this pretty quickly.

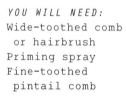

YOU WILL NEED:
Wide-toothed comb
 or hairbrush
Priming spray
Fine-toothed
 pintail comb

  #THEELLEBRAID

STEP 1 Detangle the hair and spritz with primer. Use your pintail comb to create a side parting.

STEP 2 Take a small section of hair at the front of the head and divide into three strands, just as you would do for a French braid (pages 22—23).

STEP 3 Start to braid normally by pulling the strand that is closest to the parting of the hair across the second strand (the middle one). Repeat the process by pulling the third strand (closest to the face) across the second.

STEP 4 Release strand 3 (now in the middle) and let it fall with the rest of the hair.

STEP 5 Pick up another section, preferably right underneath the forming braid, to replace strand 3.

STEP 6 Fold the new strand over strand 2.

STEP 7 Add another strand of hair to strand 1 and fold over.

STEP 8 Continue the process around the head by repeating steps 4 to 7.

STEP 9 Finish by braiding a normal braid to the end of the hair. The trick to this is to make sure to braid around the head going downwards. Here we have curved it around the head.

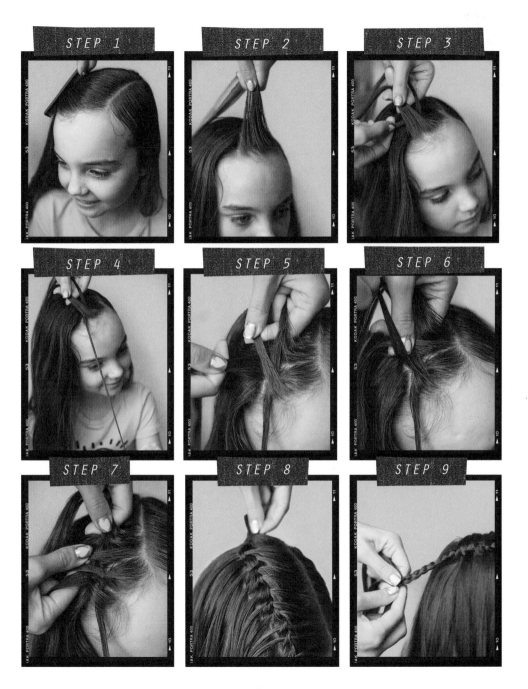

STEP 1

STEP 2

STEP 3

STEP 4

STEP 5

STEP 6

STEP 7

STEP 8

STEP 9

JOAN
JOAN

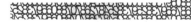

THIS TWISTED PIECE OF BRILLIANCE IS A STYLE TO BE WORN EVERY DAY OF YOUR LIFE. STAND OUT FROM THE FRENCHIES AND THE DUTCHIES WITH THIS SIMPLE FRENCH ROPE BRAID.

We named it 'Joan' after the many talented and influential Joans that have graced our planet, including Joan Smalls, Joan Crawford, Joan Didion and many others. The braid is extremely simple once you get the gist of it. Great for everyday school and sports.

  #THEJOANBRAID

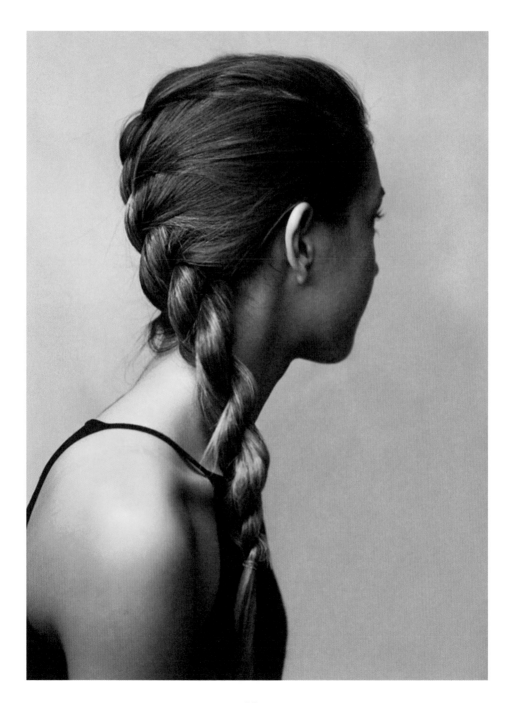

YOU WILL NEED:
Wide-toothed comb or
  hairbrush
Fine-toothed pintail
  comb
Priming spray
Water spray
Possibly an extra set
  of hands
Hair elastics

STEP 1 Detangle the hair
and spritz with primer or water
— it is a good idea to have
very damp hair for this braid.

STEP 2 To begin, take a
section from the top of the head
just as you would for a French
braid (pages 22–23). Divide this
section into three strands.
Bring the right strand over the
middle and then the left strand
over the middle.

STEP 3 Making sure that each
strand is kept separate, hold
all three in your left hand. Add
a small, even section from the
right side to the right strand.

STEP 4 Take the full right
strand; you are now going to
twist it clockwise. Keep
it tight.

STEP 5 Keep your grip
really tight and transfer
all three strands to your
right hand. Now repeat step
3 on the left side.

STEP 6 Now you must twist
the full left strand clockwise.
You may need an extra set of
hands for this part.

STEP 7 Using your left
hand, bring the twisted right
strand over to the left. The
right twist is now on the left.
The left twist is in the middle
and the other strand should be
on the right ready to have hair
added to it.

STEP 8 Repeat steps 3 to 7
until all the hair is included
in the braid.

STEP 9 Finish with a plain
Rope braid: very tightly twist
each strand and cross them
over each other.

STEP 10 Secure with an
elastic band. For extra sass
add one of our fluoro pompoms.

TIP Keep the hair wet and the
twist as tight as possible. This
is what will MAKE this braid.

STEP 2

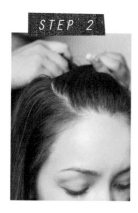

STEP 3

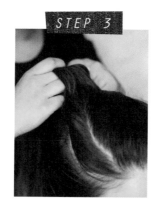

STEP 4

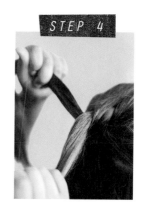

STEP 5

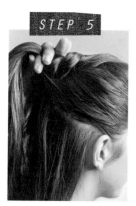

STEP 6

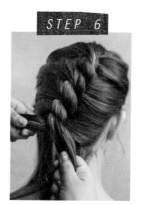

STEP 8

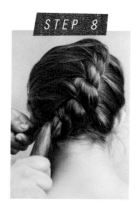

STEP 9

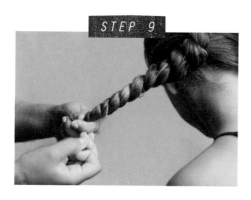

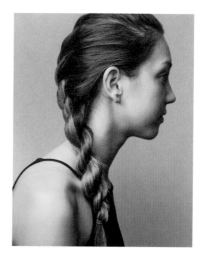

T Y

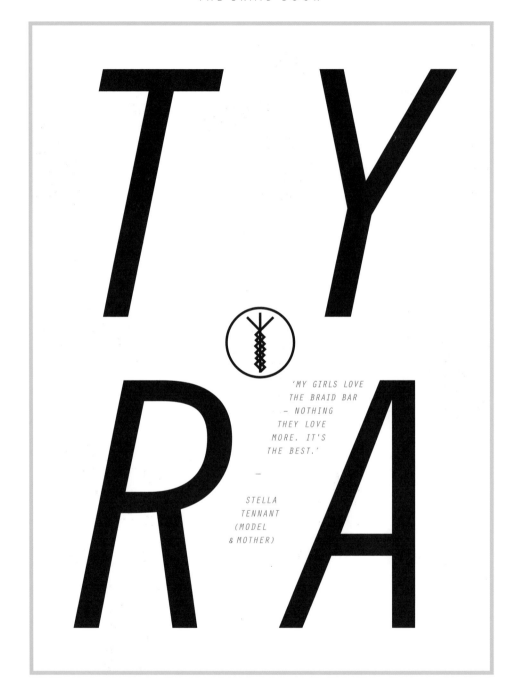

R A

'MY GIRLS LOVE
THE BRAID BAR
– NOTHING
THEY LOVE
MORE. IT'S
THE BEST.'

–

STELLA
TENNANT
(MODEL
& MOTHER)

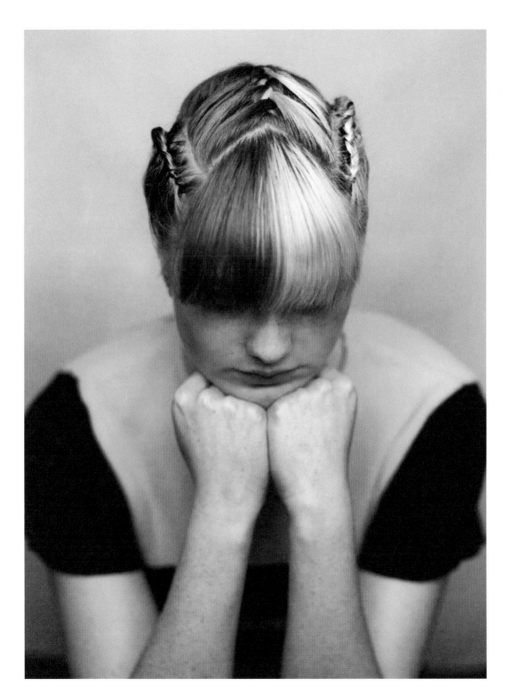

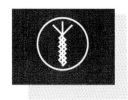

THIS IS OUR FAVOURITE OUT OF ALL THE STYLES. It is totally original and totally kick-ass! It does look complicated but if you've mastered the Lace braid and the French braid then it will be a piece of cake. No one will try to mess with you with this on your head! We called it the Tyra after the supermodel Tyra Banks because we think she's pretty kick-ass too!

YOU WILL NEED:
Wide-toothed comb
 or hairbrush
Priming spray
Fine-toothed
 pintail comb
Crocodile clip
Small elastic
 hair bands

STEP 1 Detangle the hair and spritz with primer. If you have a fringe, clip it out of the way.

STEP 2 Using your pintail comb, part the hair from the crown to the nape into three sections.

STEP 3 Clip the middle section of hair up, keeping it out of the way.

STEP 4 Start with one of the side sections, begin to Lace braid (pages 26–27) from the crown, behind the ear and all the way to the nape of the neck. Secure with an elastic band.

STEP 5 Do the same with the other side section of hair.

STEP 6 With the middle section, you may choose to do a French braid (pages 22–23) or a Dutch braid (pages 24–25). Either way, braid from the crown to the nape and secure with an elastic or clip.

STEP 7 You are now left with three sections of braided hair.

STEP 8 Split the middle into two sections. You should now have four sections of hair.

STEP 9 Proceed with a four-stranded braid (pages 28–29) to the ends of the hair and secure with an elastic band. Voilà! You are now ready to kick ass!

TOP TIP To get this braid perfect it is crucial that you are not pulling the braid too hard and that you are adding the right amount of hair as you braid. This will bring the braid closer to the centre parting rather than through the middle as a Dutch braid would look.

 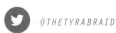
#THETYRABRAID

STEP 1

STEP 2

STEP 4

STEP 5

STEP 6

STEP 7

STEP 9

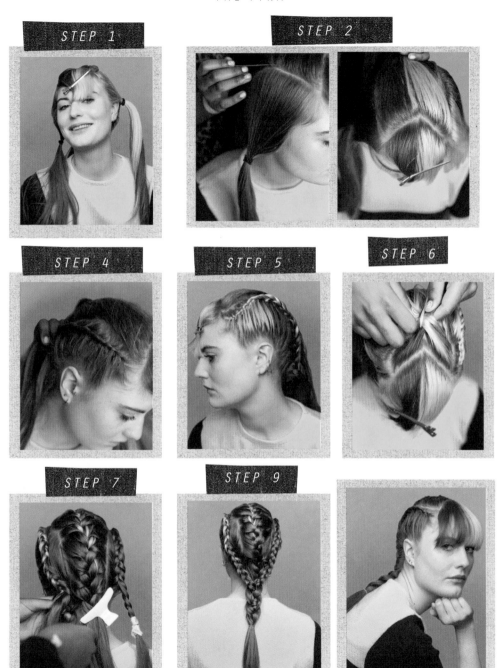

*NAMED AFTER SUPERMODEL
EVA HERZIGOVA, THIS BRAID
IS SOMETIMES REFERRED TO AS
THE 'TEMPORARY UNDER-CUT'.*

This is for all of you edgy girls who
want the look without the hassle… and
without the awkward tuft-y phase! Here
is a quick and easy way of achieving
the same look without the fear of
bringing a razor to your scalp!

EVA

EVA

EVA

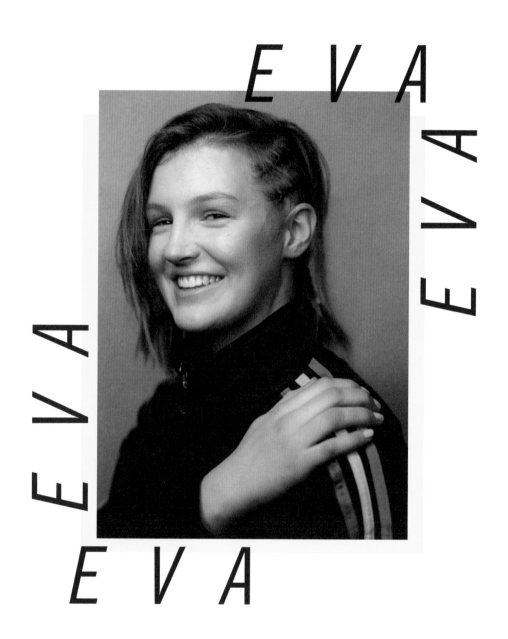

EVA

EVA

YOU WILL NEED:
Wide-toothed comb
  or hairbrush
Priming spray
Fine-toothed
  pintail comb
Hairspray

STEP 5 Now you start to form the first braid. Use the Dutch braid technique for this (pages 24–25) and whilst braiding make sure that you pull the hair very tight.

STEP 1 To create the look for this braid you will need to form two small Dutch braids, also known as cornrows.

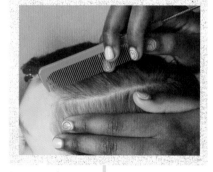

STEP 2 You need to prepare the hair by thoroughly combing it through and spritzing it with a hair primer as you do not want any loose hair in this braid.

STEP 4 The next step is to evenly separate the parting into two sections.

STEP 3 Using your pintail comb, part the hair and section above the ear in a circular shape. Make sure there is enough hair to do two braids in the section.

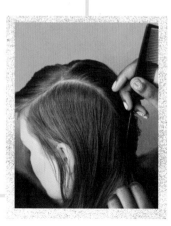

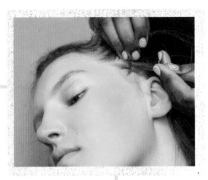

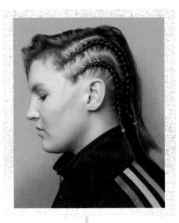

STEP 6 If you want your braids to appear as stripes, secure them at this point. If you want to continue the braid all the way down to the ends of your hair, begin to curve around the ear. Secure with an elastic band.

STEP 8 For a finishing effect, spray the hair with hairspray.

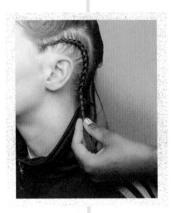

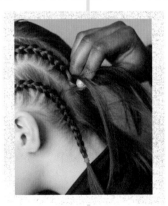

STEP 7 Repeat steps 5–6 with the other section of hair to form the second braid. Then you will see you are left with two small braids.

#THEEVABRAID

#THEEVABRAID

D O U T Z E N

THIS BEAUTIFUL STYLE IS MORE OF AN UPDO
THAN A BRAID, PERFECT FOR A WEDDING
OR SPECIAL OCCASION.

This braid is one of the simplest in the
book. We named it after Victoria's Secret
Angel Doutzen Kroes because she and the
braid seemed alike in their elegance. Add
some faux flowers and butterflies to this
braid and you are more than ready for
all your summertime events.

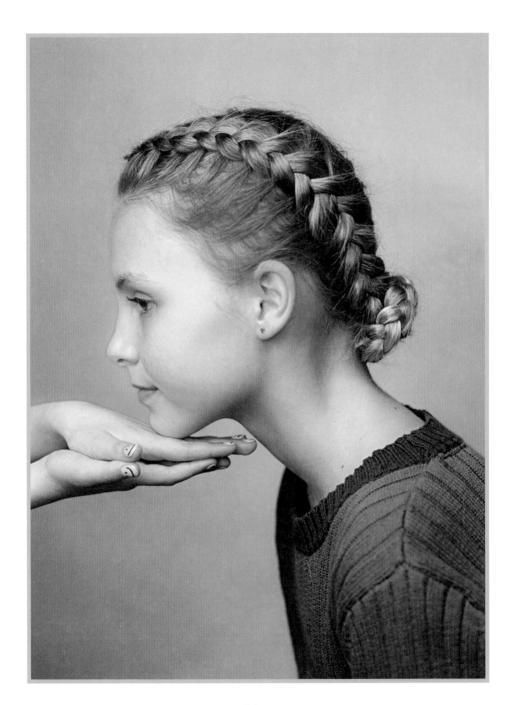

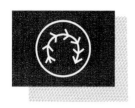

YOU WILL NEED:
Wide-toothed comb
 or hairbrush
Priming spray
Fine-toothed
 pintail comb
Elastic hair bands
Hair grips
Bristle brush,
 optional

STEP 1 Detangle the hair and spritz with primer. Pull the hair into a side parting.

STEP 2 Just as you did with the Naomi braid, begin to Dutch braid (pages 24–25) just above the inside of your eyebrow.

STEP 3 Curve the braid around towards your ear and continue it down to the nape of your neck, picking up hair from both sides of the head as you go.

STEP 4 Finish the braid with a basic plait to the ends of your hair and secure with an elastic band.

STEP 5 If your braid is quite thin, pull from both sides to loosen it.

STEP 6 At the nape of your neck, twist the braid around itself into a bun shape and secure using plenty of hairgrips.

TIPS If you want your braided bun to be thicker, add some weave (see page 19). For the perfect summer wedding look, add flowers. We found these ones on Etsy.

TRICK Using a bristle brush, gently brush along the top of your braid to get a messier look.

  #THEDOUTZENBRAID

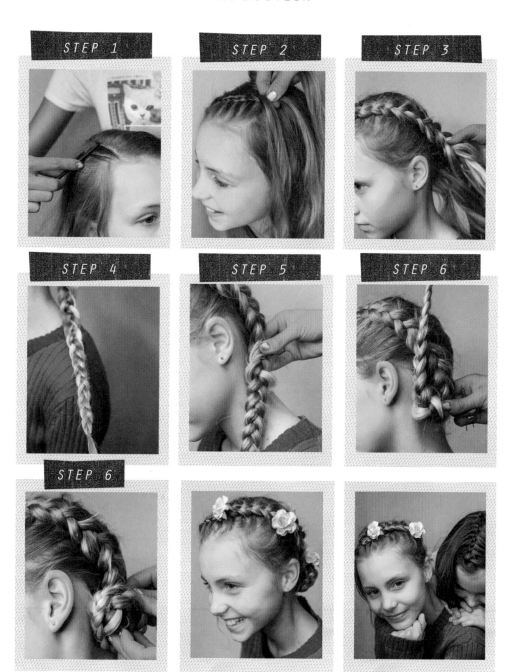

STEP 1

STEP 2

STEP 3

STEP 4

STEP 5

STEP 6

STEP 6

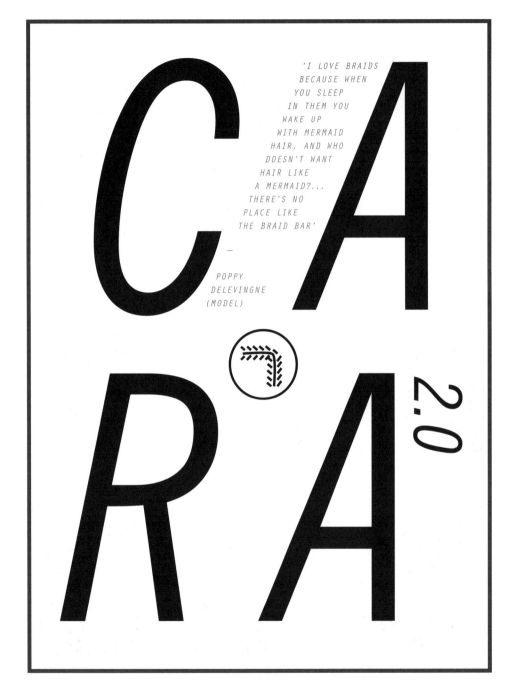

CA
RA 2.0

'I LOVE BRAIDS
BECAUSE WHEN
YOU SLEEP
IN THEM YOU
WAKE UP
WITH MERMAID
HAIR, AND WHO
DOESN'T WANT
HAIR LIKE
A MERMAID?...
THERE'S NO
PLACE LIKE
THE BRAID BAR'

–

POPPY
DELEVINGNE
(MODEL)

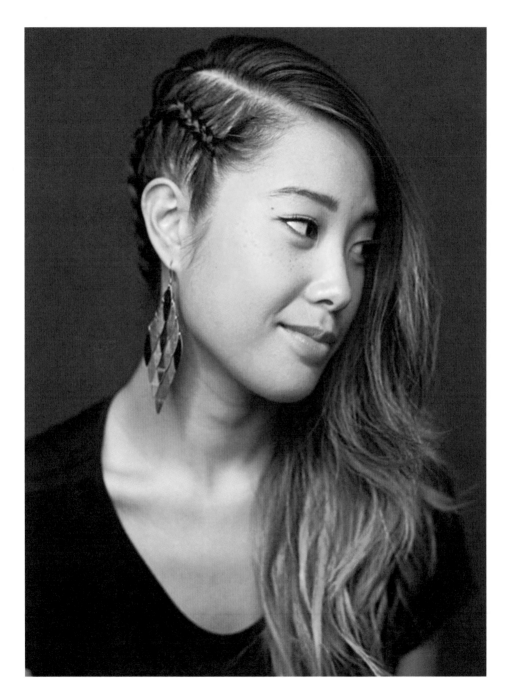

THIS BRAID BECAME FAMOUS WHEN CARA DELEVINGNE WORE IT TO THE PUNK-THEMED MET BALL IN 2013.

It is one of the most popular braids around, particularly as it works on long or short hair alike. It is basically a braided undercut that is pretty easy to do and can completely change your look with a minimum amount of fuss or effort.

YOU WILL NEED:
Wide-toothed comb
 or hairbrush
Fine-toothed
 pintail comb
Crocodile clips
Bristle brush
Hairgrips
Elastic bands
Hairspray

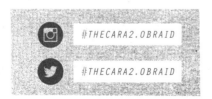

#THECARA2.0BRAID

#THECARA2.0BRAID

STEP 1 Detangle the hair and spritz with primer.

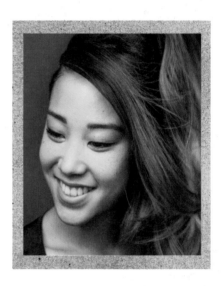

STEP 2 Using your pintail comb, make a deep parting on the side of your choice (Cara wears hers on the left side of her head). Start the parting on the hairline, directly above the arch of your eyebrow. Bring this parting to the crown of your head.

STEP 3 Once the side parting stops at the crown, continue to part the hair vertically all the way down to the nape of the neck. You should now have a third of your hair sectioned off — think of the shape of the number 7.

STEP 5 If your hair is very clean or fine, spritz the hair with a texture or volume spray. This will give your hair better grip to work with.

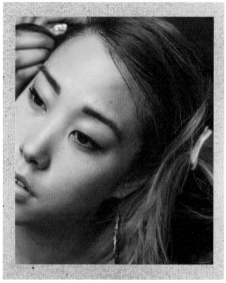

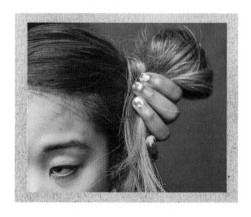

STEP 4 Leave the section of hair to braid to the side. Take the rest of your hair and clip it back.

STEP 6 For the braid: use the pin of the comb or your fingers and split the hair into three small sections right at the hairline. This is a Dutch braid, so use the basic instructions on pages 24–25 and apply them here.

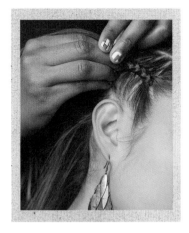

STEP 8 When you get to the nape, keep going with a regular braid (this will not be attached to the scalp). Secure with a band.

STEP 7 Curve the braid around the ear, all the way down to the nape of the neck. By this point all the hair should be included.

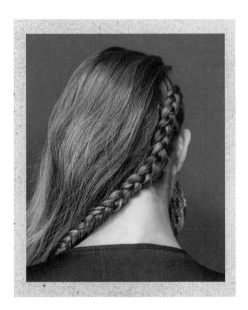

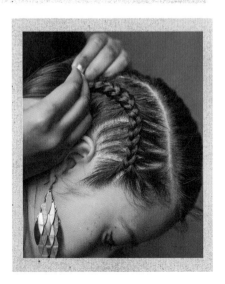

STEP 9 To finish the braid, spray with a strong-hold hairspray.

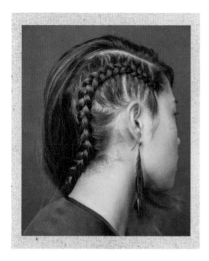

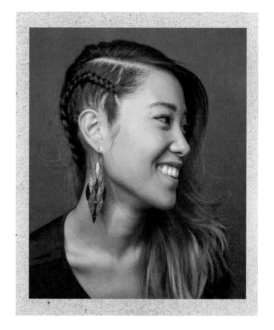

STEP 10 For the remaining hair you have several options. You might want to tong the hair, giving it some waves. You may want to blow-dry it using some volumising spray or you may want to leave it as it is, perhaps adding some sea salt spray to give it some texture.

TIP 1 If you really want to look like Cara, add an ear cuff to complete that punk look.

TIP 2 It is better to do this braid on hair that hasn't been washed for a few days.

TIP 3 This braid can be worn for a few days at a time — wash the rest of your hair as normal, just leave out the braid!

THIS BRAID IS ONE OF OUR MOST POPULAR STYLES — WE CALLED IT THE KATE AFTER OUR MOST FAVOURITE FASHION ICON, KATE MOSS.

Let's face it, she could rock any of our braids but we would love to see her with this — it's sexy, chic and a bit cheeky, just like KM! It's also great for girls who want to keep their hair down but want a different look.

If you can do a Dutch braid and you've only got ten minutes, then this is the braid for you.

It is best to do this braid on a friend or have a friend do it on you!

K A T E

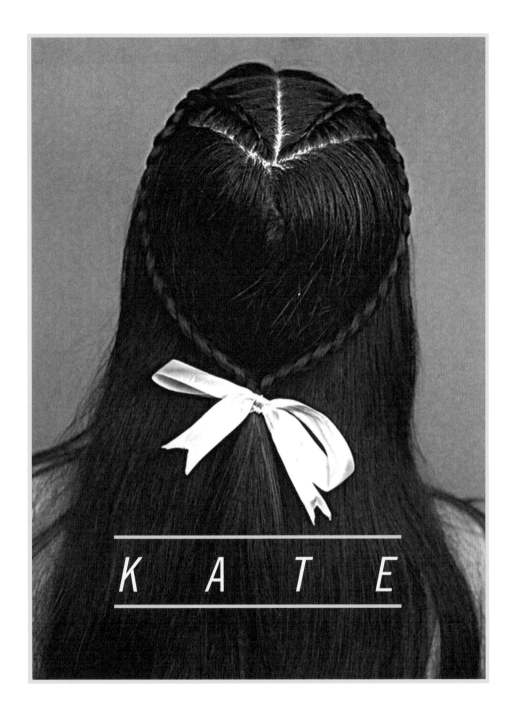

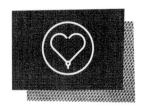

*WHY WEAR YOUR
HEART ON YOUR
SLEEVE WHEN
YOU CAN WEAR
IT ON YOUR
HEAD?*

This braid
is suitable
for most hair
types but
better on mid-
length hair.
If you have a
fringe it can
be left out or
braided in.

YOU WILL NEED:
Wide-toothed comb
 or hairbrush
Fine-toothed
 pintail comb
Crocodile clips
Hair bands
Hairspray

  #THEKATEBRAID

STEP 1 Detangle the hair and spritz with primer.

STEP 2 Using your pintail comb, part the hair down the centre.

STEP 3 Make a second parting, again using the pintail comb. Begin at the very centre of the head and part diagonally back towards the hairline creating a wedge-like shape. Pull this section of hair forward and section off. Do the same with the other side of the hair so that you are left with two equal wedges. Tie or clip back your hair below the partings made.

STEP 4 You may want to leave out the front strand of your hair. If so, do this now.

STEP 5 Take the first wedge, divide this section into three and begin doing a Dutch braid (pages 24–25). Start at the crown and curve towards the temple, then towards the back of the head, so it looks like the top curve of a heart.

STEP 6 You will not need to plait your hair to the very end as when you tie the braids together at the back, the hair below the tie is loose. This will depend on the length of your hair. Secure using an elastic band.

STEP 7 Now repeat on the other side.

STEP 8 One you have done both sides, join the ends together with a band and voilà! — you have a heartbreaker of a braid.

STEP 9 Finish off with some strong-hold hairspray to keep the braid in place and add a ribbon for cuteness or a neon band for a cool-girl look.

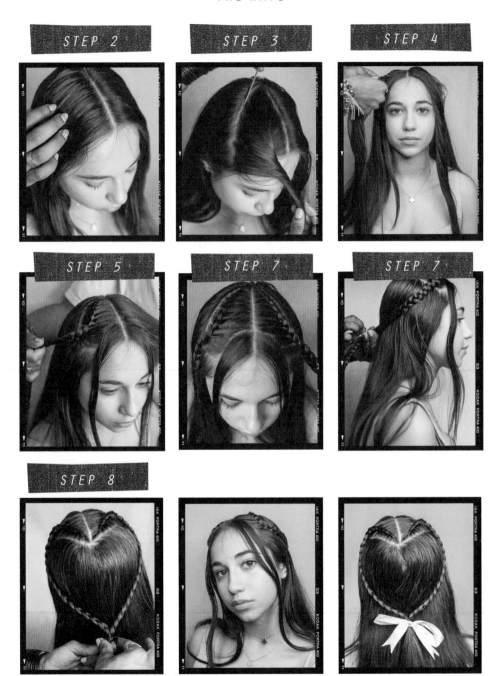

STEP 2

STEP 3

STEP 4

STEP 5

STEP 7

STEP 7

STEP 8

KEN
DALL

THIS IS NOT JUST ANY PONYTAIL, THIS IS A SEXY PONY TAIL.

This is not just a ponytail to be worn to work, this is a ponytail that you keep in after work and wear until the early hours whilst you're out partying.

This is not just any ponytail, this is The Kendall... Because it has Kendall Jenner's sophistication written all over it!

  #THEKENDALLBRAID

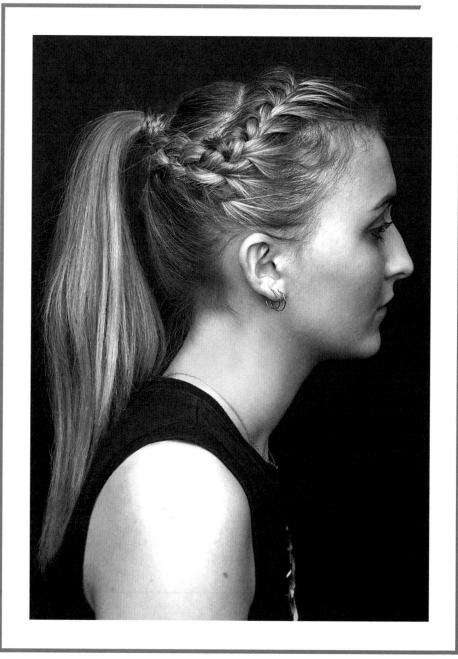

YOU WILL NEED:
Wide-toothed
 hairbrush
Priming spray
Fine-toothed
 pintail comb
Crocodile clips
Elastic hair band

STEP 1 Detangle the hair and spritz with primer.

STEP 2 Using your pintail comb, create a side parting about 5cm in length.

STEP 3 Section off the side parting by creating another parting parallel to your hairline, all the way down to your ear.

STEP 4 Clip away the hair from the side of your head and back.

STEP 5 French plait (pages 22–23) the section at the front of your head, going parallel to your hairline, starting from the side parting.

STEP 6 Follow the French plait down towards the ear.

STEP 7 Stop French braiding when you get just past the ear. Finish braiding to the end of the hair with a basic plait and secure with an elastic band.

STEP 8 Pull all the hair into a high-ish ponytail (making sure to include the braid). Remove the elastic from the braid and loosen it all out.

STEP 9 If you want to add a plait around the ponytail, take a piece of hair from underneath the ponytail, braid it using a basic plait and wrap it around the hair band for effect.

TIP When you get to the end, either cut the ribbon or tie it round the end of the braid and make a cute bow!

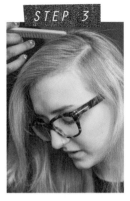

STEP 2

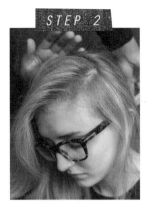

STEP 3

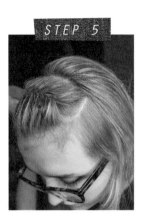

STEP 5

STEP 6

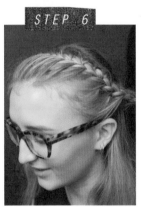

STEP 8

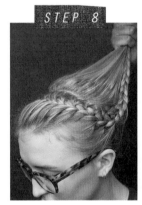

STEP 8

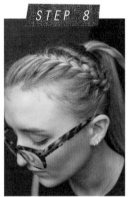

STEP 9

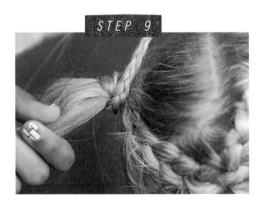

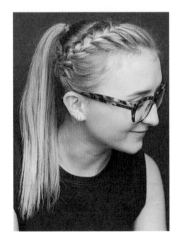

THIS IS A GREAT WAY TO UP YOUR GAME STYLE-WISE. IT REALLY ADDS SASS AND GENERAL GORGEOUSNESS TO THE STANDARD FRENCH BRAID.

We named this braid after British Olympic gold winning cyclist Laura Trott. Apart from sporting some pretty cool braids when she's racing she is an inspiration to all Braid Babes. Young, driven and unstoppable, what's not to admire?! Check out our How to French braid section (pages 22–23) before you begin.

L A U R A

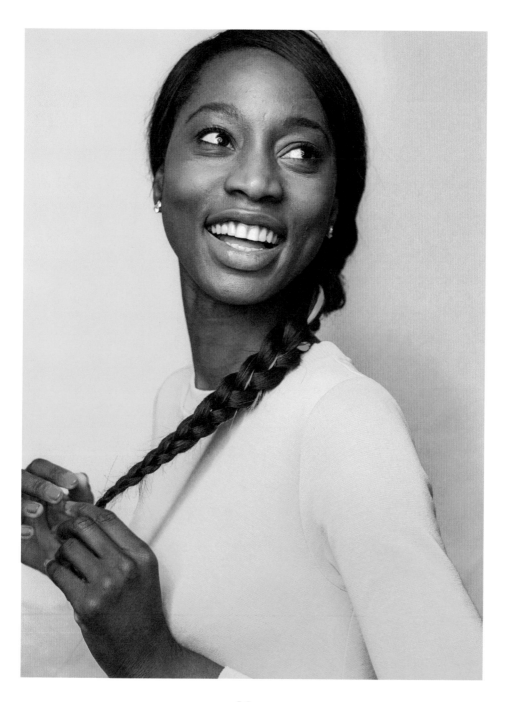

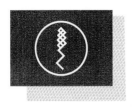

YOU WILL NEED:
Wide-toothed
 hairbrush
Priming spray
Coloured hair
 strips) or ribbon
2 hairpins
Elastic hair band

STEP 1 Detangle your hair and spritz with primer.

STEP 2 Lift a section of hair at the side of the head. Insert the hair strip or ribbon and secure with a hairpin just by the parting.

STEP 3 Divide the top hair into three sections and begin French braiding to cover the hairpin.

STEP 4 Spread the coloured hair strips and add to each part of the braid as you go. If using the ribbon, add to just one of the strands whilst you braid.

STEP 5 Be careful to adjust the ribbon to lay on top so it will be visible each time you make a new braid. When you run out of hair to add, continue with a normal braid to the end.

STEP 6 Secure with an elastic band.

TIP When you get to the end, either cut the ribbon or tie it round the end of the braid and make a cute bow.

  #THELAURABRAID

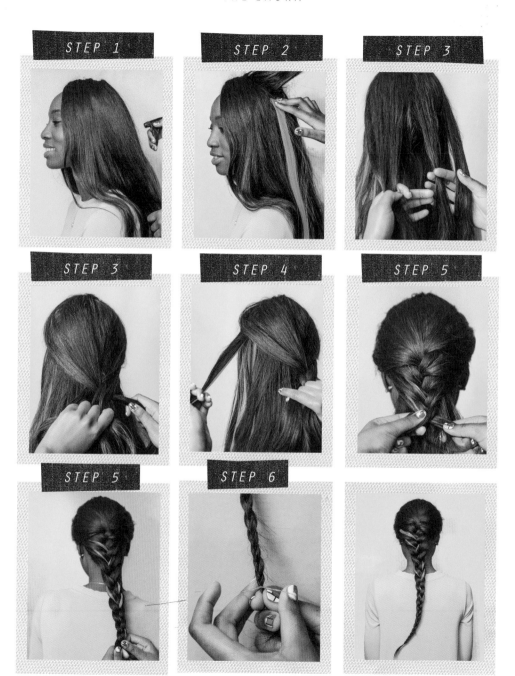

STEP 1

STEP 2

STEP 3

STEP 3

STEP 4

STEP 5

STEP 5

STEP 6

HOW COULD WE RESIST! ONE OF THE MOST INFLUENTIAL BRAID FANS OF THE MOMENT, GAME OF THRONES' KHALEESI ROCKS A DIFFERENT PLAITED STYLE EVERY EPISODE BUT THIS ONE IS DEFINITELY OUR FAVE.

This braid perfectly combines Khaleesi's power and influence with a soft and ethereal style, perfect for weddings and summer soirées. It's not too difficult either.

KHALEESI

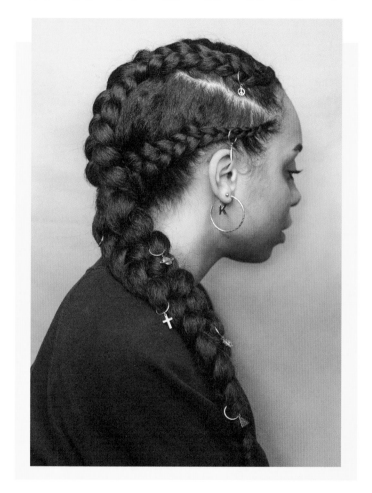

KHALEESI

YOU WILL NEED:
Wide-toothed comb or
  hairbrush
Priming spray
Fine-toothed pintail comb
Crocodile clips
Elastic hair bands

STEP 1 Detangle the hair
and spritz with primer. Using
your pintail comb, part the
hair down the centre.

STEP 2 Create a second
parting a few inches down
from the centre. Curve it
round to meet the end of
the middle parting at the
crown. Twist the hair into
a bun and clip out of the
way. This will look a bit
like a wedge shape.

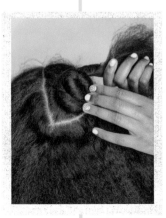

STEP 5 Repeat with
the other side of
the head.

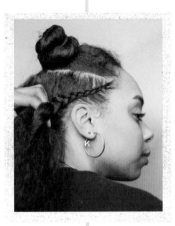

STEP 4 Begin Dutch
braiding (pages 24–25)
the side section of hair
that has been left out.
Curve the braid around
the ear and down to the
nape of the neck. Stop
at the nape and tie
with an elastic band.

STEP 3 Repeat on
the other side of
the centre parting.

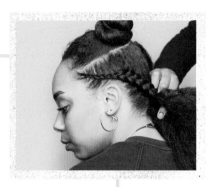

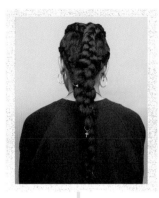

STEP 6 Now, take out one of the sections that has been clipped away. Begin to Dutch braid from the inner corner closest to the centre part and braid the outer perimeter until you reach the back. Clip away and repeat with the other half.

STEP 8 Once your braid reaches the nape of your neck, use the four-strand technique (or Dutch) and braid all the remaining hair together! Secure with an elastic band.

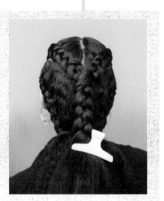

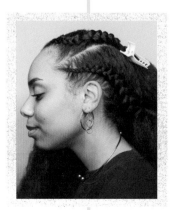

STEP 7 Once you reach the end of this section join both braids together in a Dutch braid and clip away at its halfway point.

#THEKHALEESIBRAID

#THEKHALEESIBRAID

GISELE
GISELE

*HAVE YOU ALWAYS
BEEN BAFFLED BY
THE INTRICACY OF
THE FISHTAIL BRAID?
WELL FEAR NO MORE!*

It really is one of the
easiest braids of them
all and once you get
the hang of it you'll
be so quick at it
you'll be laughing!

This step-by-step
tutorial will explain
how to do a single
fishtail braid using
all of your hair.
It really is so simple
and if you wanted to
have two fishtails
then just apply the
same process but split
the hair twice rather
than just the once.

  #THEGISELEBRAID

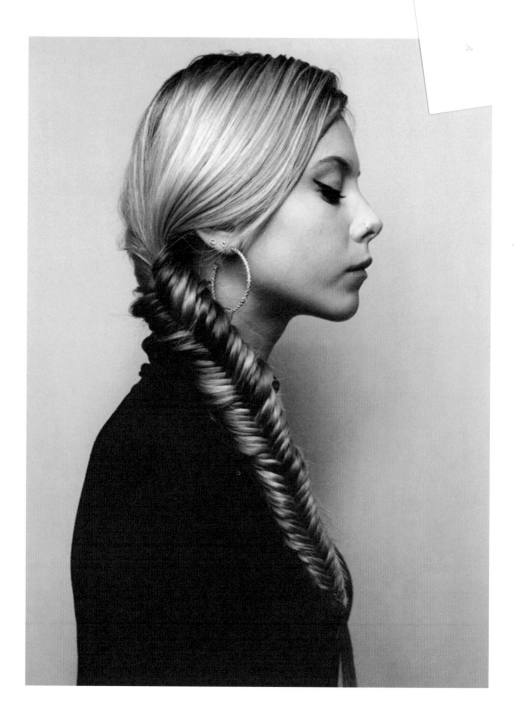

SUITABLE FOR PRETTY MUCH ALL HAIR TYPES, INCLUDING ALL THOSE CURLIER HAIRED GIRLS WHO ARE READING THIS! HOWEVER, THIS TYPE OF FISHTAIL IS DEFINITELY BETTER ON LONGER HAIR.

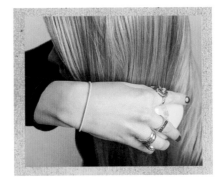

YOU WILL NEED:
Wide-toothed comb or
 hairbrush
Hair bands
Priming spray
Thickening cream
Hairspray

STEP 3 Pull all of your hair into a low ponytail at the nape of your neck. Gently tie it back with a disposable hair band (it will be cut off at the end).

STEP 1 Detangle the hair, part and spritz with primer.

STEP 2 If your hair is very clean and/or fine, it might be a good idea to use some thickening cream – this will make it easier to work with.

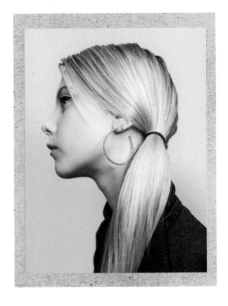

STEP 4 Divide your
ponytail into two even
sections. Unlike the
classic French or Dutch
plaits, the Fishtail
consists of only two
sections.

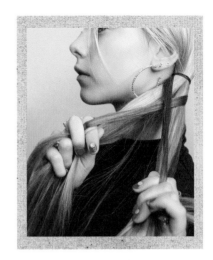

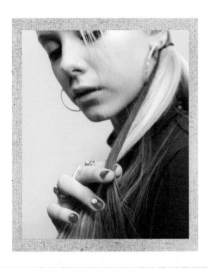

STEP 6 Continue to
pull sections from
each side. After you've
pulled each piece, re-
grip the hair to tighten
the plait but don't let
go otherwise the whole
thing will fall apart
and you will have to
start again!

STEP 5 Using your index
finger, separate a small
(not too small!) piece of
hair from the outer edge
of the right side, near the
elastic band. Pull it over
to the left side, adding
it to the opposite section
of hair. Now do the same,
taking a piece from the
left side and pulling it
over (the sections will
overlap, just the same as
they would in any French
or Dutch braid).

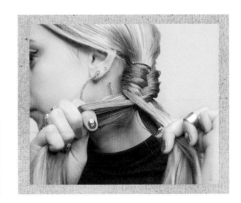

STEP 7 Once you've woven the braid to the end of your hair, use another elastic band to secure it. Now take some small but sharp scissors and carefully cut away the first elastic band.

STEP 8 If you prefer the neat, intricate look, leave the braid as it is. However, if you would like the slightly messier, effortless or ethereal look, try loosening the braid by gently tugging both sides.

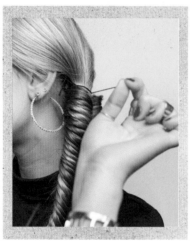

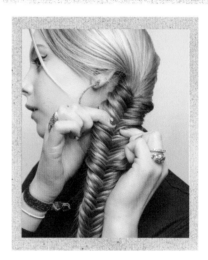

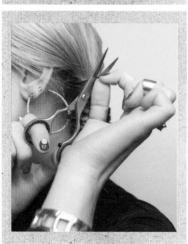

STEP 9 Final touches: finish the braid with some strong-hold hairspray — we like to use Bumble and Bumble's. Add accessories as you wish, perhaps a ribbon bow or glittery tie. Our favourite is to add one of our neon pompoms to give the look a bit more edge.

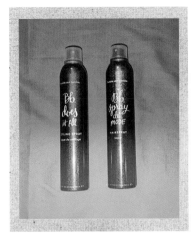

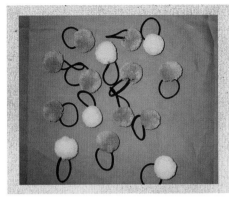

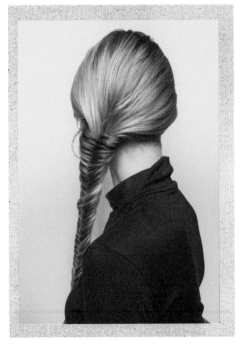

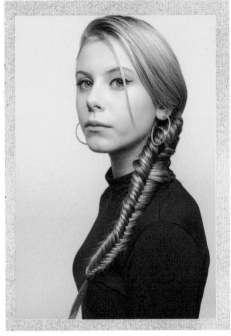

CLAUDIA

THE ULTIMATE HALO BRAID!

Inspired by the angelic Claudia Schiffer,
this is perfect for those who love all their
hair up and out of their face! This braid
is also perfect for those of you hunnies
with a fringe as it looks fabulous when
left out of the plait.

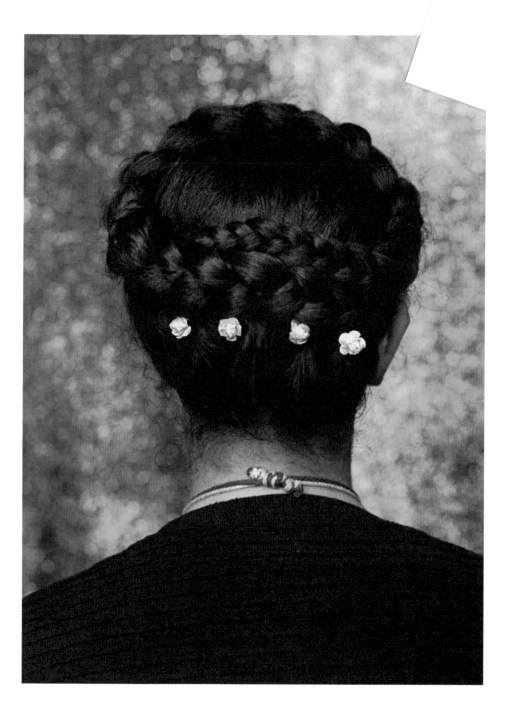

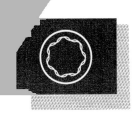

YOU WILL NEED:
Wide-toothed comb
 or hairbrush
Priming spray
Texturising or
 salt spray
Fine-toothed
 pintail comb
Crocodile clip
Small elastic
 hair bands
Hairgrips
Hairspray

STEP 1 Detangle the hair and spritz with primer.

STEP 2 If you have very fine or soft hair then it may be a good idea (once detangled) to use a texturising spray — for example, a salt spray.

STEP 3 Using your pintail comb, start by parting the hair from ear to ear over the crown of the head, leaving more hair at the back.

STEP 4 Clip away the front of the hair.

STEP 5 Start Dutch braiding (pages 24–25) from behind the ear — pick up three strands of hair and start to braid parallel to the hairline.

STEP 6 You need to add hair as you go along and when you bring the hair into the braid make sure that you brush it, so you get a smooth result rather than lots of lumps and bumps.

STEP 7 Carry on braiding around the head and take your time because the more you braid, the more hair is involved.

STEP 8 Once the braid meets with the beginning again, carry on braiding the hair off the scalp and pin it to join the rest of the braid using a hairgrip.

STEP 9 Use hairspray to finish and add accessories for added style.

  #THECLAUDIABRAID

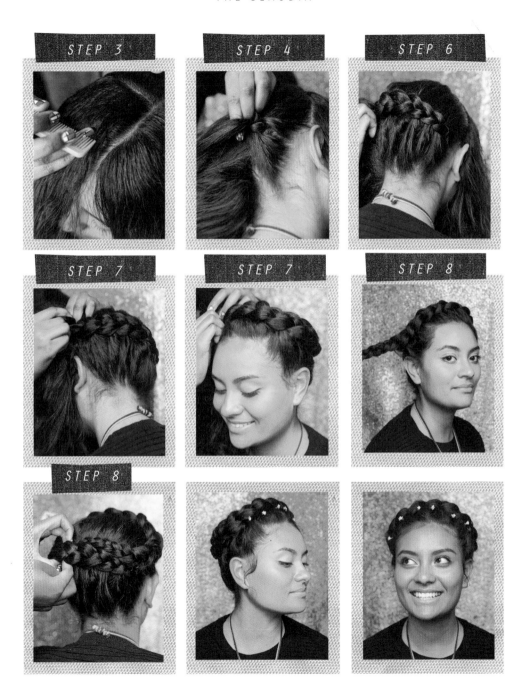

STEP 3

STEP 4

STEP 6

STEP 7

STEP 7

STEP 8

STEP 8

THIS IS A PERFECT LOOK FOR SCHOOL OR THE OFFICE, IT LOOKS PRIM FROM THE FRONT AND ROCKING FROM THE BACK.

We named this one after Christy Turlington as she is the perfect supermodel — she's super slick and has that 'All American girl' look, but we reckon she's a tiger underneath!

We think this style is best on quite long hair as the buns need a bit of volume, but if you're willing to tease your hair before then you could give it a go on any length hair.

CHRISTY

YOU WILL NEED:
Wide-toothed comb or
 hairbrush
Priming spray
Fine-toothed pin-tail comb
2 elastic hair bands
Hairpins
Hairspray

STEP 5 Do a standard braid with each section and secure with a band.

STEP 1 Detangle the hair and spritz with primer.

STEP 2 Part the hair in the middle with your comb, all the way down the head so you have two equal sections on both sides.

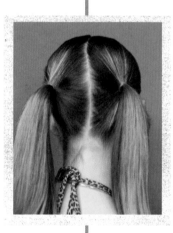

STEP 4 Tie each section into ponytails, making sure they are even.

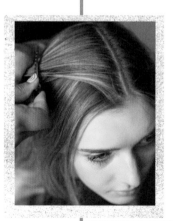

STEP 3 Smooth the hair down — make it nice and tight.

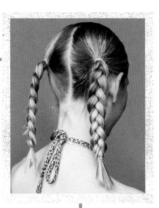

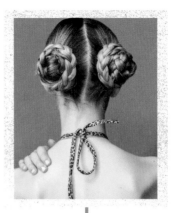

STEP 6 Loosen the braids by pulling on both sides.

STEP 7 Wrap one braid around itself to form a bun and use plenty of hairpins to secure.

TIP: If your hair isn't quite long enough, add some weave (page 19). You can either braid it in or braid a section of extra hair and wrap around each bun and secure with hairpins, as we have done here.

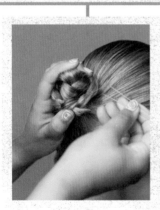

STEP 10 Add a heap load of hairspray and you're ready to go. Pretty easy, huh?

STEP 9 Give the head a bit of a shake when you've finished just to make sure you've fastened the buns to the head securely.

STEP 8 Repeat on the other side.

#THECHRISTYBRAID

#THECHRISTYBRAID

LINDA

 #THELINDABRAID

 #THELINDABRAID

WE NAMED THIS BRAID AFTER SUPERMODEL LINDA EVANGELISTA.

Like her, it's elegant, smart and sophisticated. Perfect for the office, school or ballet class! We love this braid as it can be smart but a bit sassy at the same time — from the front you mean business and from the back you're all about the fun!

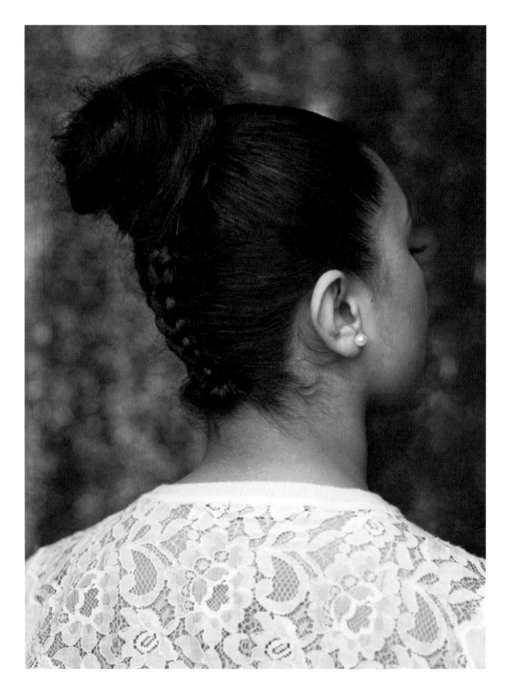

YOU WILL NEED:
Wide-toothed comb
 or hairbrush
Priming spray
Fine-toothed
 pintail comb
Crocodile clips
Elastic hair
 band
Hairpins
Strong-hold
 hairspray

STEP 1 Detangle the hair and spritz with primer.

STEP 2 Using your pintail comb, part the hair from ear to ear. Clip away the top half.

STEP 3 Flip your head over and brush your hair towards the floor so all your hair is upside down.

STEP 4 Dutch braid (pages 24–25) from the nape of the neck upwards, making sure to keep the braid in the centre.

STEP 5 Stop Dutch braiding when you get to the crown of the head. Use a basic braid to the end of the hair and tie using an elastic band.

STEP 6 Spritz with some more primer, if needed.

STEP 7 Take the front section of the hair out and pull all the hair together (including the braid) and tie up on the top of your head like a high ponytail.

STEP 8 Twist the hair around the base to form a bun and pin to hold.

TIP 1 If your hair is very thin, backcomb to create volume.

TIP 2 If you're wearing this to work or school, make sure you give it a good spray with some strong-hold hairspray.

TIP 3 You may want to wear it out after work, so simply add some glitter and hair chalk for sassiness!

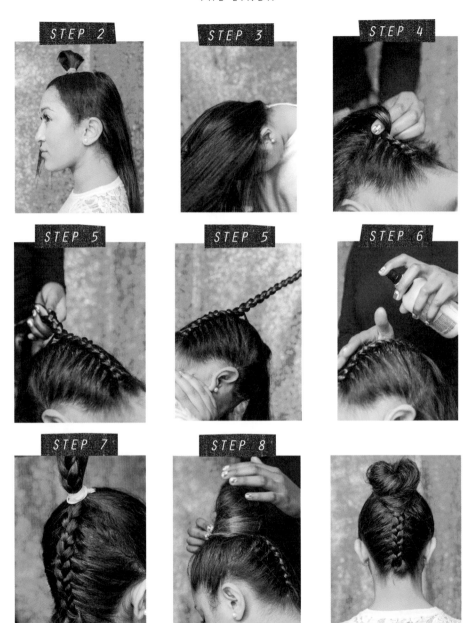

STEP 2

STEP 3

STEP 4

STEP 5

STEP 5

STEP 6

STEP 7

STEP 8

GWEN

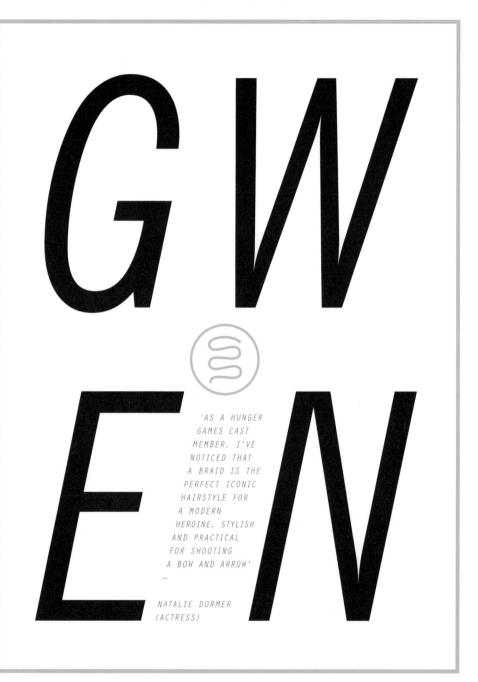

'AS A HUNGER
GAMES CAST
MEMBER, I'VE
NOTICED THAT
A BRAID IS THE
PERFECT ICONIC
HAIRSTYLE FOR
A MODERN
HEROINE. STYLISH
AND PRACTICAL
FOR SHOOTING
A BOW AND ARROW'
—

NATALIE DORMER
(ACTRESS)

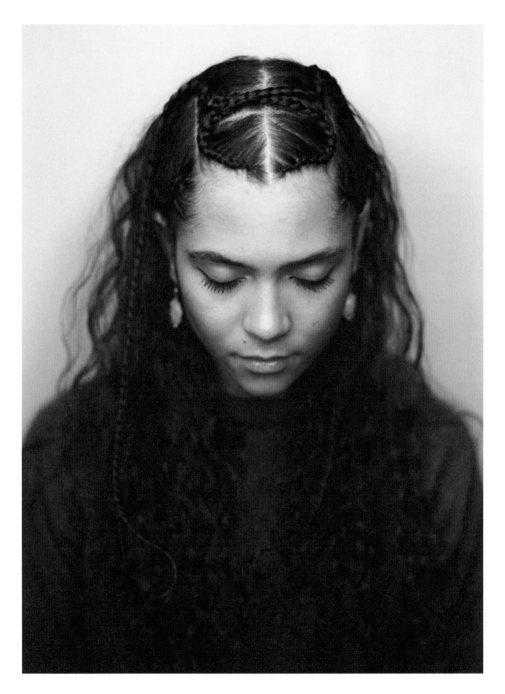

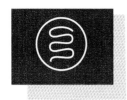

NAMED AFTER THE ONE AND ONLY GWEN STEFANI - possibly one of the coolest women in the world. This braid represents Gwen in her 1990s days and it's safe to say it is one of our more complicated braids. This is definitely one of the best styles to wear for a festival. It is edgy, cool and your hair will be out of your face for all that dancing you'll be doing!

YOU WILL NEED:
Wide-toothed comb
  or hairbrush
Priming spray
Fine-toothed
  pintail comb
Small elastic
  hair bands
Crocodile clip
Hairspray

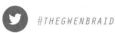
#THEGWENBRAID

STEP 1 Detangle the hair and spritz with priming spray — it will be easier to do this on slightly damp hair.

STEP 2 Using the pintail comb, divide the hair from ear to ear and tie away the rest of the hair.

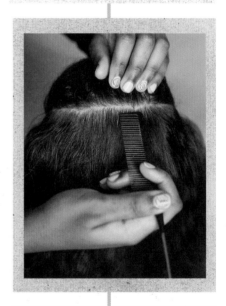

STEP 3 Now divide the front section into three parts, with the middle section larger than the two side sections.

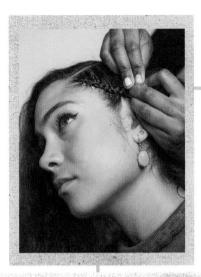

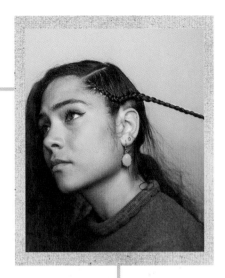

STEP 4 Starting with one side, Dutch braid (pages 24–25) following the curve of the ear, then braid to the end. Secure with an elastic band.

STEP 5 Do the same with the other side section.

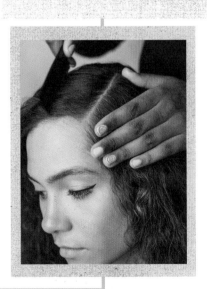

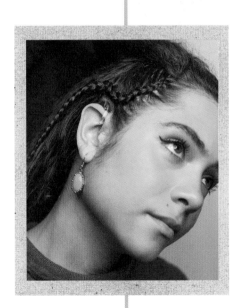

STEP 6 You now need to divide the middle section of hair into four quarters, one parting down the centre, and one horizontally across.

STEP 10 Bring the plait down and continue to Dutch braid, collecting the hair from the top of square 3, around the perimeter of the square to the bottom right corner.

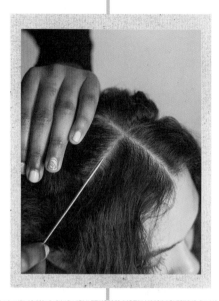

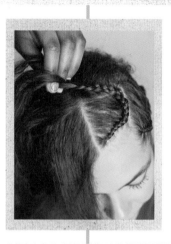

STEP 9 Lift the braid from the scalp and plait the hair until it reaches square 3's top right corner.

STEP 7 Let's number the squares 1 to 4 going clockwise. Clip squares 2 and 4 away, focusing on 1 and 3.

STEP 8 Begin with square 1 and Dutch braid from the top right corner around the perimeter, forming a curved right angle.

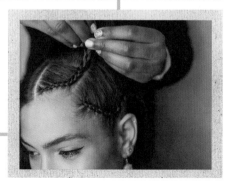

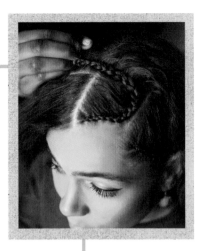

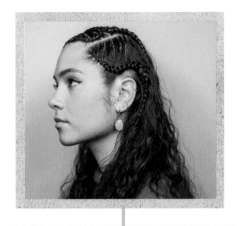

STEP 13 Hairspray
to finish!

STEP 11 Repeat with
squares 2 and 4 starting
with the top left corner of
square 2 and Dutch braiding
around its perimeter
creating a right angle,
lifting the plait until it
reaches the top left corner
of square 4 and Dutch
braiding down the square's
perimeter to the bottom
left corner.

STEP 12 We like to finish
with basic braids to the
end of the hair. Secure
with an elastic band.

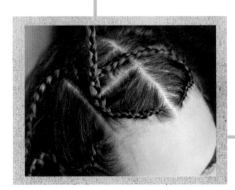

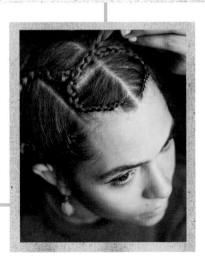

*PREVIOUSLY 'THE CARA' WE HAVE RENAMED
THIS BRAID AFTER OUR BRAND AMBASSADOR
MADDI WATERHOUSE.*

Younger sister of Suki, Maddi is a rising
star and the perfect idol for you hunnies.
This is a half up/half down style; this is
probably why it is so popular at The Braid
Bar. I don't think you'll see it anywhere
else — it's a sort of mash up between the
Kate and the Naomi. We love to add charms to
it to give it a bit of an edge (Suki would
definitely approve!) but it looks super cool
without too. Check out My Flash Trash charms
or Regal Rose charm rings to see what
we're talking about!

MADDI

*'THE BRAID BAR IS THE COOLEST. WHAT'S NOT TO LOVE?
GET INSPIRED AND BECOME A PUNK, A PRINCESS, HIPPIE
— WHATEVER YOUR STYLE INSPIRATION IS.'
SUKI WATERHOUSE (MODEL)*

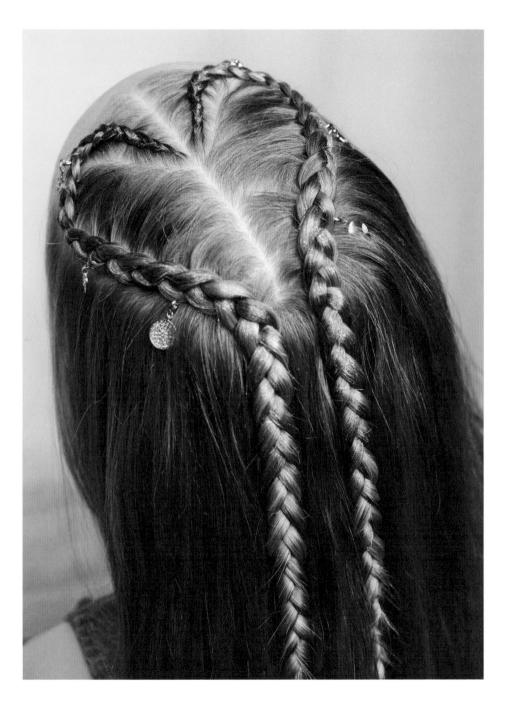

YOU WILL NEED:
Wide-toothed
 comb or
 hairbrush
Priming spray
Fine-toothed
 pintail comb
Crocodile clip
Small elastic
 hair bands

STEP 1 Detangle the hair and spritz with primer.

STEP 2 Part the hair down the centre from the hairline to the crown.

STEP 3 From the crown end of the parting, make another parting diagonally towards the temple. Repeat on the other side.

STEP 4 Clip or braid the rest the hair out of the way.

STEP 5 Starting from the top of the small triangle, Dutch braid towards the front of the head.

STEP 6 Curve the braid as you go, rotating it back to the edge of the bigger triangle and braid the hair around its perimeter until you reach the back of the triangle.

STEP 7 At the crown of the head, stop Dutch braiding and finish with a basic plait to the end of the hair. Secure with an elastic band.

STEP 8 Repeat on the other side.

  #THEMADDIBRAID

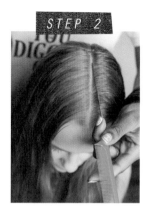

STEP 2

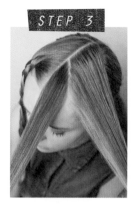

STEP 3

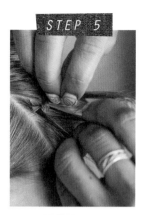

STEP 5

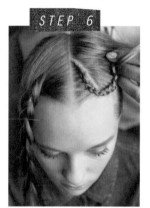

STEP 6

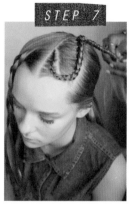

STEP 7

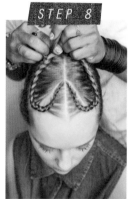

STEP 8

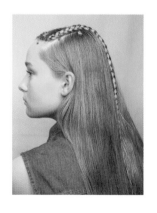

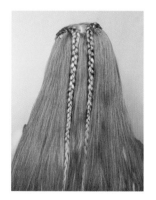

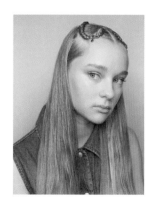

NOW THIS IS MAJOR! WE HAVE
SAVED THE BEST TO LAST — THIS IS
DEFINITELY FOR ALL YOU BRAID FANS
WITH ENDLESS AMOUNTS OF HAIR.

We called this style the Heidi after
supermodel Heidi Klum. Like our braid,
she is a lot of pretty cool things all
rolled into one — supermodel, mum,
TV star and underwear designer
— a power braid babe!

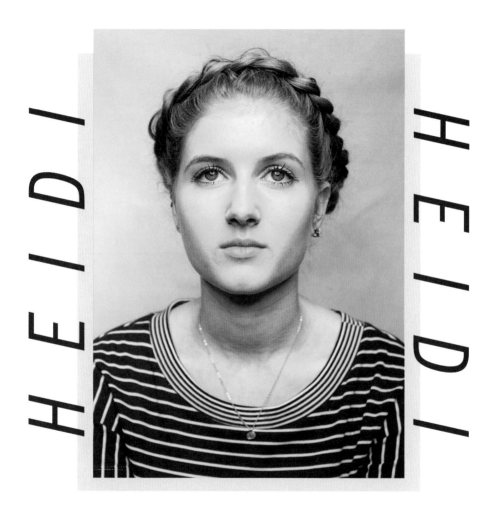

HEIDI

HEIDI

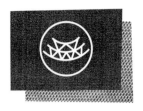

YOU WILL NEED:
Wide-toothed comb
 or hairbrush
Priming spray
Fine-toothed
 pintail comb
Crocodile clips
Elastic hair bands
Hairgrips
Hairspray

  #THEHEIDIBRAID

STEP 1 Detangle the hair and spritz with primer.

STEP 2 Using your pintail comb, make a parting about 2.5—5cm in from the hairline, all the way around in a semicircle.

STEP 3 Part again from underneath, just on the crown of the head and clip away the rest of the hair underneath and to the side.

STEP 4 You should be left with a semicircle shape in the middle of the head. Gather all the hair in this section and proceed to Dutch braid (pages 24—25) from the right, curving the braid around the parting in a circular shape.

STEP 5 You should eventually make a circle shape and end up back at the ear on the side that you started.

STEP 6 Carry on braiding, adding the hair from around the ear as you go, travelling all around the back of the head until you reach the nape on the furthest side.

STEP 7 Finish the braid with a basic plait and secure with an elastic band.

STEP 8 Once the braid is finished, pull on the sides to loosen it and give it that dishevelled effect.

STEP 9 Turn the end of the braid on itself and secure it between the other braids, using lots of hairgrips.

STEP 10 Secure with hairspray.

TIP This braid is best for people with lots and lots of long hair!

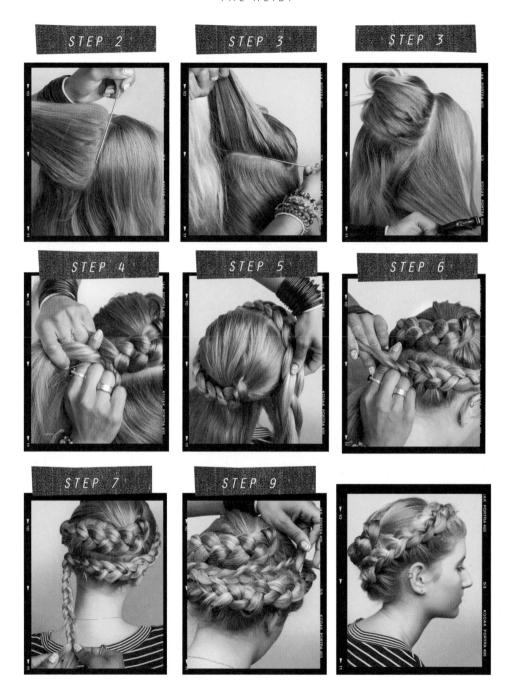

STEP 2

STEP 3

STEP 3

STEP 4

STEP 5

STEP 6

STEP 7

STEP 9

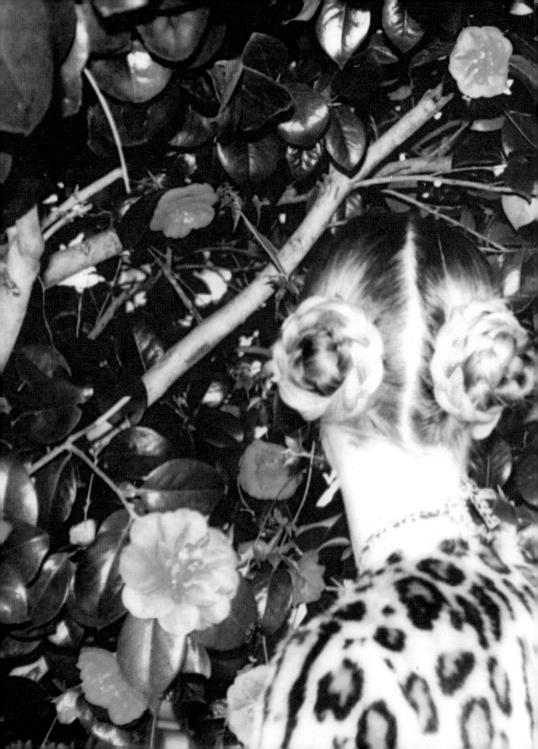

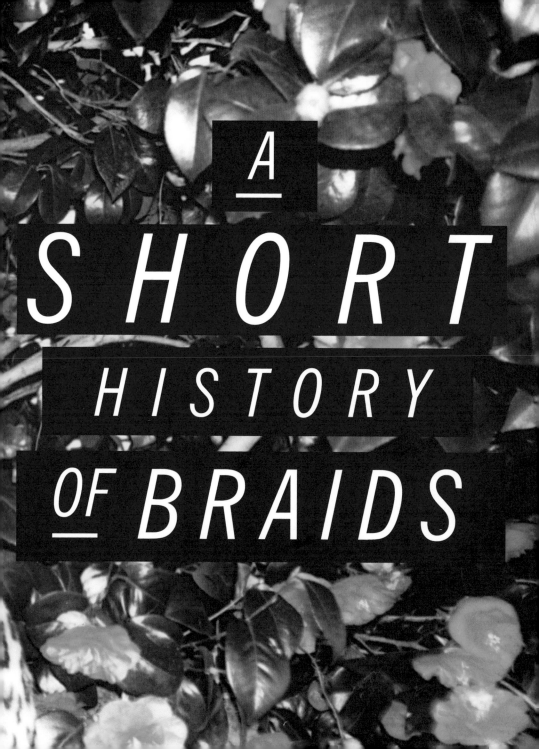

A SHORT HISTORY OF BRAIDS

DID YOU KNOW THAT MOST BRAIDING STYLES DATE BACK TO ANCIENT TIMES?

HERE ARE SOME FACTS ABOUT THE HISTORY OF ANCIENT BRAIDS…

AFRICAN BRAID

• Braiding is an ancient form of decorating hair that is widespread in Africa and worn as both a cultural trait and a fashion statement.

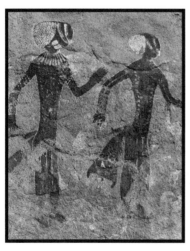

TASSILI N'AJJER ROCK PAINTING

• The earliest depiction of cornrows is thought to be a rock painting in the Tassili n'Ajjer plateau of the Sahara in Algeria, dating from 3000 BC. The different styles can be used to identify tribe, religion, kinship, marital status, age, ethnicity, wealth and status.

• Despite many Africans having their hair cut short when sold into slavery and transported overseas, the tradition survived and made its way to Europe and America, possibly as an act of defiance.

• From the 1920s, when straightening methods improved, the cornrow lost some popularity with African-American women. However, they remained popular with children.

• Styles vary from straight to rounded to complex geometric braids. More elaborate patterns are traditionally worn for special occasions such as weddings, ceremonies and war preparations. The patterns are usually handed down through generations.

• The women of the Himba tribe in Namibia paint their braids with an ointment made from red

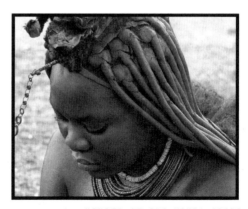

MEMBER OF THE HIMBA TRIBE

ochre, butter, ash and herbs. The Masai tribes in Tanzania and Kenya also prefer red hues and dye their hair this colour.

FRENCH BRAID

- Although its name suggests this braid originated in France, it actually originates from Africa, as with cornrows. In the several thousand years since, it also became popular with the early Greeks, Celtic nobles and during the Chinese Song dynasty period (960–1297). It was first referred to as 'French' in the American Arthur's Home Magazine in 1871, but it's unclear why.

" ... DO
UP YOUR
HAIR
IN THAT
NEW
FRENCH
BRAID ... "

DUTCH BRAID

- Also called an 'inverted French braid', this braid is believed to have originated in Holland. It is similar to the French braid, though new hair is

added under rather than over the braid. It also has close similarities to cornrows, which are also made close to the head. This method is popularly used to create a circular 'crown' around the head.

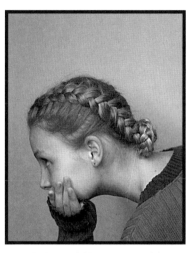

THE DOUTZEN (PAGES 60–63) USES A DUTCH BRAID

SWISS BRAID

- Made popular by the book Heidi, this is a circular braid worn around the head like a crown (similar to Grecian styles) and made using the Dutch braid method.

FISHTAIL BRAID

- Originated in the 19th century when it was referred to as a 'Grecian braid'. Also known as Herringbone braid.

A FEW OTHER STYLES...

EGYPTIAN BRAID

- As in Elizabeth Taylor's depiction of Cleopatra, ancient Egyptians (both men and women) with social standing braided their hair into mini braids all over the head. Recently Blake Lively has demonstrated a take on this style with a few 'peek-a-boo' braids.

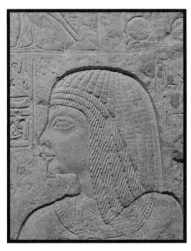

HEIROGLYPH DEPICTING A WOMAN

CHINESE QUEUE BRAID

- During the Qing dynasty (1644-1912), men from Manchuria shaved off all hair above their temples and plaited the remaining hair into a long pigtail or Queue. Not wearing the Queue was considered treason until 1922, when the last emperor of China cut his off, declaring the style no longer in fashion.

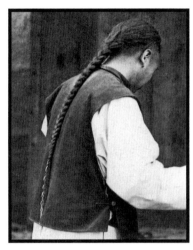

CHINESE MAN WITH QUEUE BRAID

CELTIC BRAID

- Ancient Celtic knots and braids date back to 700 BC. Noblewomen and men would wear their hair long, braiding it into elaborate designs and those in the lower classes would wear simpler knots at the top of their head to keep hair out of their eyes.

GRECIAN BRAID

- Upper-class women in Ancient Greece would braid their hair (or have their hair braided by servants) into spirals around the hairline and all over the head. Servants and slaves wore shorter haircuts and subsequently did not wear braids, so they were a demonstration of social standing.

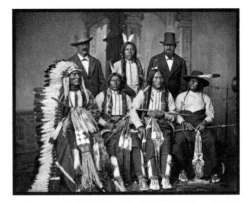

NATIVE AMERICANS IN TRADITIONAL DRESS

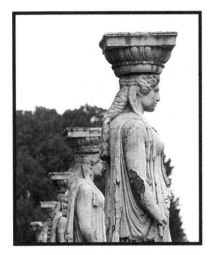

CARYATTDS AT VILLA ADRIANA

MEDIEVAL BRAID

- Older noblewomen were required to cover their hair in the Middle Ages to avoid accusations of being witches, so they wore tight, braided crowns from which they hung headpieces.

NATIVE AMERICAN BRAID

- The origin of pigtails can be traced back to Native American tribes. Each of the (more than 500) tribes in North America had different styles, decorating with ribbons, deerskins, etc. Similar to African braiding, the type of braid worn determines social and marital status and identity.

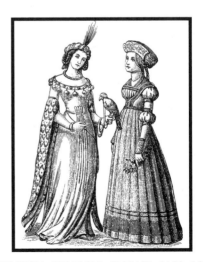

MEDIEVAL EUROPEAN FASHION 1450-1500

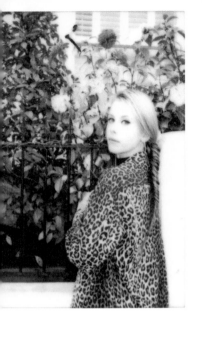
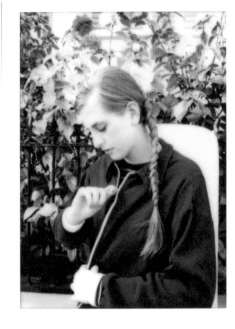
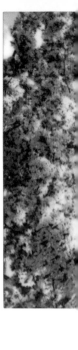
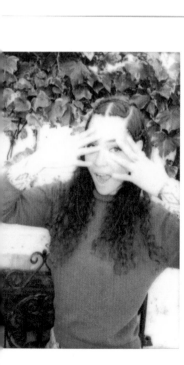
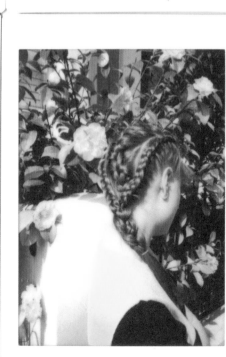
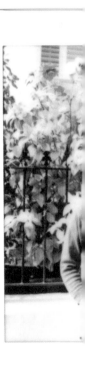

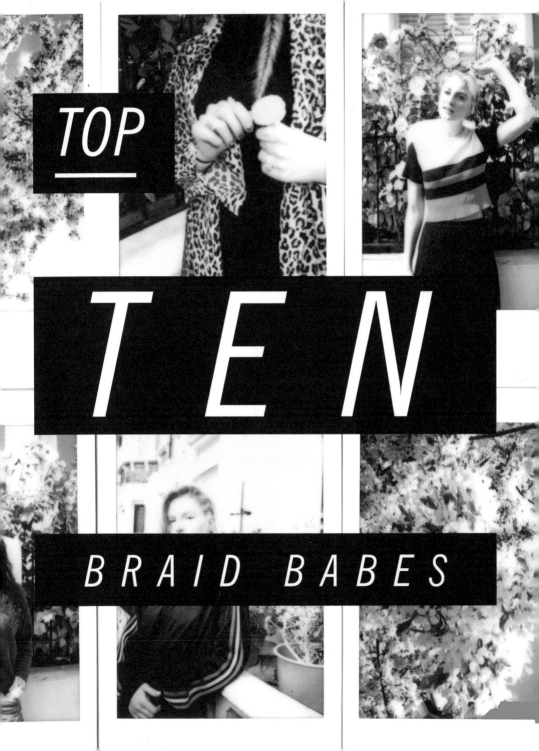

TOP

TEN

BRAID BABES

1. CLEOPATRA

Well she had to be our number one! Not only beautiful but a kick-ass queen to boot — no one messed with her or her braids!

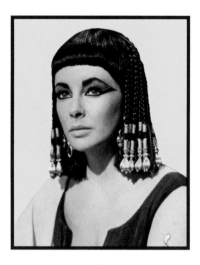

2. BEYONCÉ

Is there anything we don't love about her? She knows how to rock a good braid more than anyone!

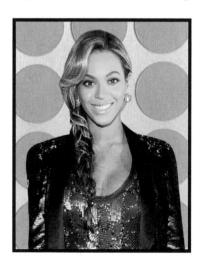

3. LUPITA NYONG'O

This Oscar-winning actress's favourite pastime is braiding with her best friends. Wish we were one of them!

4. KHALEESI

She introduced braids to a whole new audience — not only that but showed us medieval braids rock!

5. LAURYN HILL

When she released 'Killing Me Softly' in 1996, Lauryn was rocking a long braided style — and we've loved her ever since.

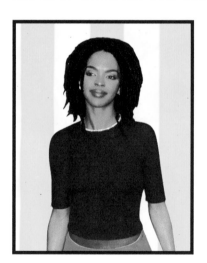

6. GWEN STEFANI

Always reinventing herself, she managed to bring cultures together and wore cornrows with absolute style.

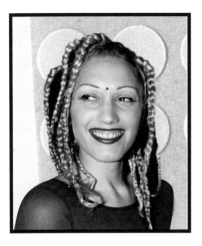

7. HEIDI KLUM

Thank you Heidi for giving us the supremely sexy but also the ultimate 'don't mess with me' braid. You are our cowgirl dream!

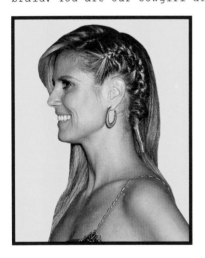

8. ELSA

We couldn't possibly have a top ten braid babe list without our Frozen superstar. When it comes to a braid, Elsa showed us how to 'Let It Go!'

9. CARA DELEVINGNE

When she turned up to the Met Ball with her braided undercut she proved yet again what an original she is.

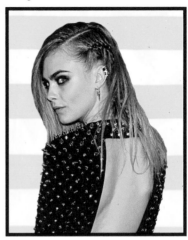

10. ALICIA KEYS

We've saved the best till last! Alicia burst on to the music scene in 2001 rocking braids and beads. We 'Keep on Fallin' for her bold and beautiful style.

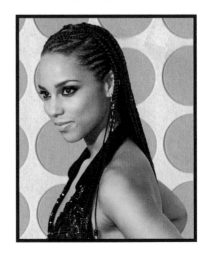

ACKNOWLEDGEMENTS

A huge thank you to everyone at Kyle, especially Claire Rogers for her patience and tolerance with Willa and me — all those endless emails and phone calls! Thank you to Lotte and Jo for the amazing design — they have made the book look super cool and without their vision it would have looked rubbish! And Jesse Jenkins for taking the beautiful photos! Thank you Jenny Dyson and her pencils for making The Braid Bar look like The Braid Bar. Thank you Bay Garnett for all her help and support, tirelessly helping us with quotes and lending us her style and sass. Thank you to all of our incredible models, our make up artistes Celia Burton and Lucy Pearson, our nail guru Kione Grandison, and Nicola Easton for providing delicious food on the shoots.

And finally and most importantly, we want to thank our families: Renshaw, Linus, Bache and especially Lucy, who gave Sarah the idea for The Braid Bar; and Nicola, Matthew and Celia.

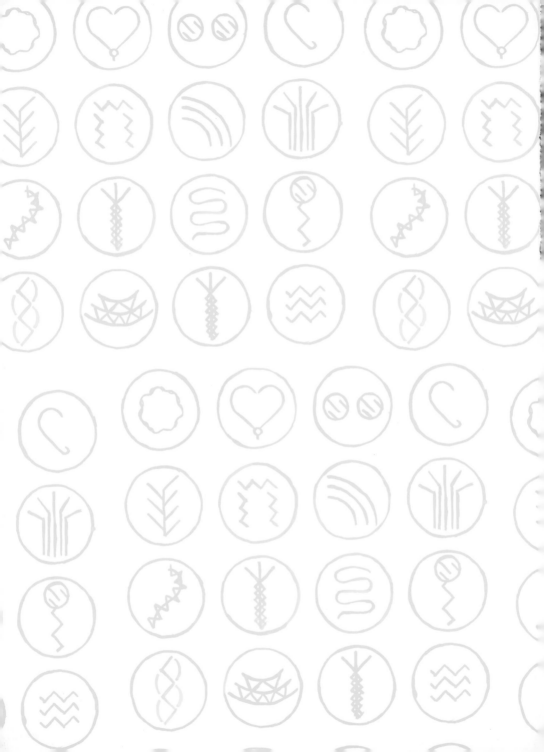